A History of American Neurology

A History of
American Neurology

Russell N. DeJong, A.B., M.S., M.D.

Professor Emeritus of Neurology
The University of Michigan Medical School
Ann Arbor, Michigan

Raven Press ▪ New York

Raven Press, 1140 Avenue of the Americas, New York
New York 10036

Great care has been taken to maintain the accuracy of the information
contained in the volume. However, Raven Press cannot be held responsible
for errors or for any consequences arising from the use of the information
contained herein.

DeJong, Russell N.
  A history of American neurology.

  Includes bibliographies and index.
  1. Neurology—United States—History. I. Title. [DNLM: 1.
Neurology—History—United States. WL 11 AA1 D3h]
RC339.A1D4   616.8′0973   80-6270
ISBN 0-89004-680-8   AACR2

To Madge, and to Mary, Connie, and Russ

Preface

This volume, a detailed study of the development of neurology as a science and a medical discipline in the United States, focuses on the backgrounds as well as the accomplishments of the many American physicians and scientists who have contributed to our knowledge of the nervous system. It is intended to provide the reader with a fascinating and informative account of the noteworthy events that have occurred in American neurology.

The first three chapters trace the early evolution of American neurology. These chapters discuss the establishment of neurology as a special discipline in American medical education and medical practice, the close association between neurology and psychiatry, the significant discoveries of the men who are known as the fathers of American neurology—Silas Weir Mitchell and William Alexander Hammond—and the founding of the American Neurological Association. The middle chapters of the book emphasize specific persons who have made important contributions to the field of neurology in the latter part of the 19th century and in the 20th century. These include such well-known neurologists as Bernard Sachs, Harvey Cushing, Derek Denny-Brown, and Houston Merritt. The next few chapters cover the rapid expansion of clinical neurology in the 20th century. These chapters detail the advances made in the diagnosis of diseases of the nervous system, the evolving concepts of the etiology and pathophysiology of such disorders, and the new and more effective therapeutic approaches to them. The text concludes with chapters on neurologic organizations and publications and on neurology in the federal services, including the Armed Forces, the Veterans Administration, and the United States Public Health Service.

This book, written principally for students and practitioners of clinical neurology and of the neurosciences, is directed also to readers with a general interest in medical history.

Acknowledgments

Through the kindness of Stanley A. Nelson, I was given the opportunity to review the proceedings of the History Committee of the American Academy of Neurology, as recorded over many years. Richard J. Allen contributed historical material about the Child Neurology Society. *The Centennial Anniversary Volume of the American Neurological Association,* edited by Derek Denny-Brown, A. S. Rose, and A. L. Sahs, was an important source book, as was *The Nervous System,* edited by Donald B. Tower, which was written to celebrate the twenty-fifth anniversary of the National Institute of Neurological and Communicative Disorders and Stroke.

I am grateful for the assistance of my secretary, Bart MacMillan; the staffs of the Michigan Historical Collections in the Bentley Historical Library and the A. Alfred Taubman Medical Library, both at the University of Michigan; and the editorial staff at Raven Press.

Contents

A History of American Neurology

1

American Medicine Prior to the Development of Neurology as a Specialty

As was the case in most countries of the western world, American neurology and psychiatry originated and developed in the early years as a dual medical specialty. Later, however, during the first few decades of the second half to the nineteenth century, neurology became a separate entity in the United States and western European countries, especially in Germany, France, and England.

MEDICINE DURING THE NINETEENTH CENTURY

Modern medicine evolved gradually during the first half of the nineteenth century (11). With the introduction of new diagnostic tools and methods, improvements were seen in the clinical examination. Percussion of the chest as a diagnostic procedure had been described by Leopold von Auenbrugger in 1751, but his discovery was ignored and the procedure remained unnoticed until 1808 when it was revived by Baron Jean Nicolas Corvisart. The stethoscope was invented in 1819 by René Théophile Hyacinthe Laennec, who published his *Traité de l'auscultatione médiate* the same year. Sir John Floyer described counting the pulse using a watch in 1707, but this also was ignored and did not come into general use until the 1830s and 1840s when it was introduced by Pierre Charles Alexandre Louis in France and William Stokes in Ireland. General anesthesia with ether was first utilized by Crawford W. Long in 1842, but he failed to publish an account of it. It was not until 1846 that the first published reports appeared describing ether anesthesia given by William Thomas Green Morton to patients operated on by John Collins Warren.

During the first part of this century there were a number of contributions to neurology (20). Andrew Marshall published *The Morbid Anatomy of the Brain in Mania and Hydrophobia* in 1815 (19), and John Cooke (1756–1838) published *A Treatise on Nervous Diseases* in 1820 (5); the latter consisted of three sections, "On Apoplexy," "On Palsy," and "On Epilepsy." Sir Charles Bell (1774–1842) published *The Nervous System of the Human Body* in 1830 (1). Marshall Hall (1790–1857) published *Lectures on the Nervous System and Its Diseases* in 1836 (12); and François Magendie (1783–1855) published *Leçons sur les fonctions et les maladies du systeme nerveux* in 1839 (18). The first significant advances in clinical neurology, however, were to await the contributions of Romberg and Duchenne.

Many more techniques and tools, now considered essential to medical diagnosis and treatment, were described during the second half of the century (11). The ophthalmoscope was invented in 1851 by Hermann von Helmholtz. In 1865 Gregor Johann Mendel established the principles of inheritance, and 2 years later Joseph Lister (soon to become Lord Lister) published two papers describing and recommending aseptic surgery. Although the first treatise on thermometry had been published in 1740 by George Martine, no clinical and scientific basis for the technique was established until 1868, when Carl Reinhold August Wunderlich did so. Thermometers were beginning to appear in hospitals in 1866 and 1867, but the early ones were 10 inches long, and a period of 5 minutes was required to determine the axillary temperature. The pocket thermometer was introduced by Sir Clifford Allbutt in 1868. Hugo Kronecker and Ritter von Basch carried out the first sphygmomanometric studies on human beings in 1878, but determination of the systolic and diastolic blood pressures was not described until 1896 by Scipione Riva-Rocci. During the 1870s, Pasteur, Koch, and others established the microbial etiology of many diseases, and in 1895 Wilhelm Konrad Roentgen discovered what he termed the X-ray.

DEVELOPMENT OF NEUROLOGY IN WESTERN EUROPE

During the latter half of the nineteenth century, while clinical neurology was emerging as a medical specialty in America, three major schools of neurology developed in Europe, in Germany, France, and England. These should be mentioned because they evolved simultaneously with neurology in America and because the American version of neurology was significantly influenced by that in Europe. At the forefront of the German School was Moritz Romberg (1795–1873), professor of neurology and director of the University Hospital in Berlin. He studied in Vienna and began his career in neurology by translating into German Andrew Marshall's *The Morbid Anatomy of the Brain* in 1820 and Sir Charles Bell's *The Nervous System of the Human Body* in 1831. His own classic text *Lehrbuch der Nervenkrankheiten des Menschen,* which was published in parts from 1840 to 1846, was the first systematic treatise on clinical neurology and was a major milestone in the development of this specialty. It was translated into English in 1853 by the Sydenham Society (25). Among Romberg's students and followers were

Heinrich Erb, Nikolaus Friedreich, Hermann Oppenheim, Adolf van Strumpell, and Karl Wernicke.

The first of the famous French neurologists was Amand Duchenne (1806–1875), who practiced first in Boulogne and then in Paris. The real flowering of French neurology, however, took place during the time of Jean Martin Charcot (1825–1895), who was chief physician at the Salpêtrière and was appointed professor of diseases of the nervous system in the Faculty of Medicine of the University of Paris in 1882. He was the master of the French School, and his students, associates, and followers included Edme Felix Alfred Vulpian, Joseph Jules Dejerine, Joseph Francois Babinski, Pierre Marie, and others.

Neurology gained prominence in England with the establishment of the National Hospital for the Paralyzed and Epileptic in Queen Square, London in 1860, where the first physicians were Jabez S. Ramskill and Charles Édouard Brown-Séquard. However, more significant advances were made later, by John Hughlings Jackson (1835–1911), William Richard Gowers (1845–1915), and David Ferrier (1843–1928) (6,15).

THE REVOLUTIONARY WAR AND DEVELOPMENT OF MEDICINE AS A PROFESSION

There were no medical schools in the United States prior to the Revolutionary War, nor were there medical specialties. Practitioners of medicine were trained by serving as apprentices to older physicians, or preceptors, thereby learning their methods of practice. The more affluent and more ambitious would-be physicians received their education at the prominent medical centers in Europe, principally those in Edinburgh, London, Paris, and Leiden. Medicine was established as a profession in the United States during the Revolutionary War. In fact, the war played an important role in establishing the careers of the three leading physicians of the time—John Morgan (1735–1789), William Shippen, Jr. (1706–1808), and Benjamin Rush (1745–1813), all educated in Europe.

Morgan, with the collaboration of Shippen, established the first medical school in this country (10), the College of Philadelphia, in 1765. This became the Medical Department of the University of Pennsylvania in 1791. By 1800 there were four medical schools in the United States: one at the University of Pennsylvania; one at Kings College in New York City, which was established in 1765; one in Boston, the Harvard Medical School, which was opened in 1782; and one in Hanover, New Hampshire, the medical school of Dartmouth College, which was opened in 1798. The medical school of Kings College was taken over by the College of Physicians and Surgeons, and this in turn became the medical department of Columbia University in New York City.

EARLY AMERICAN REFERENCES TO DISEASES
OF THE NERVOUS SYSTEM

In the early days there were no medical specialties, and each physician engaged in the practice of all aspects of medicine. Neurology, if practiced at all, was carried out by the general physician, and psychiatry was generally neglected. Some of the early physicians, however, had a definite interest in diseases of the nervous system and made contributions to our knowledge of them. James Jackson (1777–1868), the first physician to the Massachusetts General Hospital and maternal grandfather of James Jackson Putnam, in his *Letters to a Young Physician Just Entering Upon Practice* discusses the nervous system, headaches, epilepsy, apoplexy, palsy, chorea, neuralgia, pain, and insanity (17). He also provided one of the earliest descriptions of alcoholic neuritis. John Ware (1795–1864), professor of the practice of medicine at the Harvard Medical School from 1832 to 1858, made an exhaustive study of delirium tremens. John Kearlsy Mitchell (1798–1858), the father of S. Weir Mitchell, was an eminant physician and teacher and had a deep interest in diseases of the nervous system. Robley Dunglison (1798–1869) compiled an excellent medical dictionary and wrote an amazing array of medical textbooks covering almost every aspect of medicine. In his two-volume *Practice of Medicine* he included a section of 175 pages on diseases of the nervous system (8). Daniel Hosack (1769–1835) the best known practitioner in New York City in his time, had an interest in diseases of the nervous system, as did Theodore Romeyn Beck (1791–1855), author of *Elements of Medical Jurisprudence* (1823), which went through many editions. Beck also served, from 1849 to 1854, as the second editor of the *American Journal of Insanity*.

Internal medicine gradually developed as a specialty, and many of the leading internists had a continuing interest in the nervous system and its diseases. Included here are such physicians as Austin Flint, Sr. (1812–1886) and Abraham Jacobi (1830–1919) of New York, Jacob N. DaCosta (1833–1900) of Philadelphia, and William Osler (1849–1919) of Philadelphia and Baltimore. This interest continued into the succeeding generation of internists, and such physicians as Lewellys F. Barker and William S. Thayer also made contributions to neurology.

EARLY CONTRIBUTIONS TO KNOWLEDGE
OF THE NERVOUS SYSTEM

Neurology had its beginnings as a specialty in the United States at the time of the Civil War (1861–1865), and the impetus for its development is the result of the work of two men, Silas Weir Mitchell (1829–1914) and William Alexander Hammond (1828–1900). There are three men, however, who made significant contributions to what was to become America's neurology specialty before the time of Mitchell and Hammond. Two of these were psychiatrists, but, as noted, neurology and psychiatry developed together in America as well as in most European countries, and it is difficult to establish just when their separation began. Mitchell and Hammond practiced and contributed to psychiatry as well as neurology, even though they called themselves neurologists. This is true also for the next few generations of neurologists. The third man was not an American and was more of a neurophysiologist than a neurologist, although he called himself both; he actually was in America for only short periods of time.

Benjamin Rush (1745–1813) is claimed by psychiatrists to be the "father of American psychiatry," but his name should also be included in a discussion of the development of American neurology (Fig. 1) (2,7,9,10,21,24). Rush belonged to that group of versatile individuals who helped bring about the independence of the United States. He was one of the signers of the Declaration of Independence, was a member of the Constitutional Congress, and was appointed Treasurer of the United States Mint in 1797 by President John Adams. His major contributions, however, were in the field of medicine, where he served as practitioner and teacher. He began his training in medicine as an apprentice to Dr. John Redman, at that time the leading physician in Philadelphia, and then entered the University of Edinburgh, from which he received his medical degree in 1768. He then returned to Philadelphia, where he became one of the eminent physicians of his time, although many of his principles (e.g., bloodletting as a mode of treating almost every illness) had no scientific rationale (27). He was appointed professor of the theory and practice of medicine in the College of Philadelphia in 1789 and became professor of the Institutes of Medicine and Clinical Medicine in the Medical School of the University of Pennsylvania when the College of Philadelphia merged with that school in 1791. He was physician to the Pennsylvania Hospital and established a ward for the treatment of mental patients there in 1756.

The most comprehensive course in mental disease in America was taught by Rush, and in 1812, the year before his death, he published what was probably his most important scientific work, *Medical Inquiries and Observations Upon the Diseases of the Mind,* the fifth in his cyclopedic series of *Medical Inquiries and Observations* (Fig. 2) (26). The majority of Rush's opinions and conclusions on the diagnosis and the treatment of mental disease were derived from his personal observations in the Pennsylvania Hospital where he was in charge of the care of mental patients for more than 30 years. He had few authorities upon whom he could rely when making his statements, for no texts in psychiatry had been published in this country at that time, and even in Europe there had been none of importance. His book went through many editions and served for several decades as the primary textbook and standard reference work for American practitioners and students of mental disease. For many years it was the only American textbook

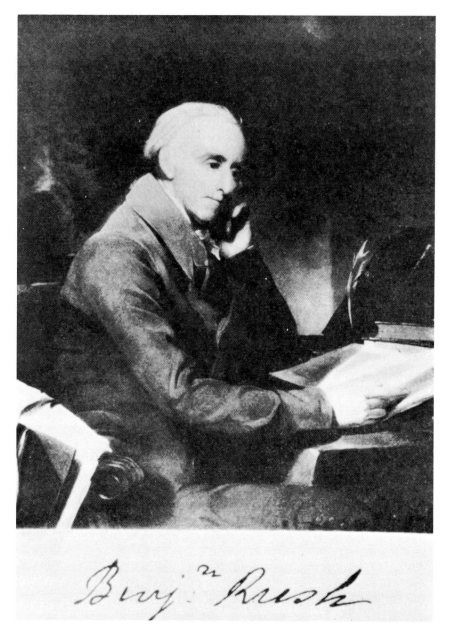

FIG. 1. Benjamin Rush. Portrait by Benjamin Sully, in the Pennsylvania Hospital. (From ref. 7)

MEDICAL INQUIRIES

AND

OBSERVATIONS,

UPON

THE DISEASES OF THE MIND

BY BENJAMIN RUSH, M. D.
Professor of the Institutes and Practice of Medicine, and of Clinical
Practice, in the University of Pennsylvania.

PHILADELPHIA:

PUBLISHED BY KIMBER & RICHARDSON,

NO. 237, MARKET STREET.

Merritt, Printer, No. 9, Watkin's Alley

1812.

FIG. 2. Title page of Rush's *Medical Inquiries and Observations Upon the Diseases of the Mind.*

on psychiatry. Isaac Ray's *Medical Jurisprudence of Psychiatry* was published in 1838, but it dealt with only one phase of the subject. It was not until 1883, when Hammond's *A Treatise on Insanity and its Medical Relations* was published, that any outstanding contributions to the field of psychiatry had been made or any other systemic treatise on mental disease was available (13). Hammond had, prior to this, published a small book (77 pages) dealing with one aspect of psychiatry, *Insanity in Its Relation to Crime* in 1873 (14). Spitzka's book *Insanity, Its Classification, Diagnosis and Treatment* appeared in 1883 (28).

Rush believed that mental disease was primarily the result of congestion and inflammation of the blood vessels, with extension of the morbid process to the nerves and to that part of the brain, considered to be the seat of the mind. He classified the causes of mental diseases into two groups: One consisted of those acting directly on the body or the brain, in which he included injuries to the brain, tumors, apoplexy, and epilepsy. The others were those acting on the body or the brain through the medium of the mind.

The other early American psychiatrist who also made contributions to the understanding of diseases of the nervous system was **Amariah Brigham** (1798–1849) (Fig. 3) (16). He was one of the 13 founding members of the Association of Medical Superintendents of American Institutions for the Insane in 1844, which was to become the American Medico-Psychological Association in 1894, and finally the American Psychiatric Association in 1921. Also, in 1844 he founded the *American Journal of Insanity,* which later became the *American Journal of Psychiatry,* and served as its editor until his death 5 years later.

Brigham, born in New Marlboro, Massachusetts, served an apprenticeship under Dr. Edmund C. Peet of New Marlboro and then completed his medical education by taking a course of lectures at the College of Physicians and Surgeons in New York City. He first practiced general medicine and surgery, and then turned to psychiatry; in 1840 he was appointed superintendent of the Retreat for the Insane in Hartford, Connecticut, and in 1842 he was appointed superintendent of the State Lunatic Asylum in Utica, New York, where he remained until his premature death. During the year of his appointment at Hartford he published the first American book dealing with neurology, *An Inquiry Concerning the Diseases and Functions of the Brain, Spinal Cord, and Nerves* (Fig. 4) (3). In the preface he called the attention of those practitioners of medicine into whose hands his book might fall to the importance of the nervous system and tried to persuade them to embrace every opportunity for studying its functions and diseases. He discussed the structure and functions of the brain, medulla, spinal cord, and cranial nerves. Although most of the clinical portions of the book deal with mental diseases, he did discuss inflammation of the brain, apoplexy, epilepsy, tinnitus, chorea, delirium tremens, and tic douloureux.

Charles Édouard Brown-Séquard (1816–1894) was a peripatetic neurologist and neurophysiologist (Fig. 5) (22,23). He spent much of his time traveling between the island of Mauritius, France, England, and the United States. It was said that he crossed the Atlantic Ocean more than 60 times. He was born on Mauritius, the son of a French mother (Charlotte Séquard) and an American sea captain who was lost at sea prior to Charles' birth. He

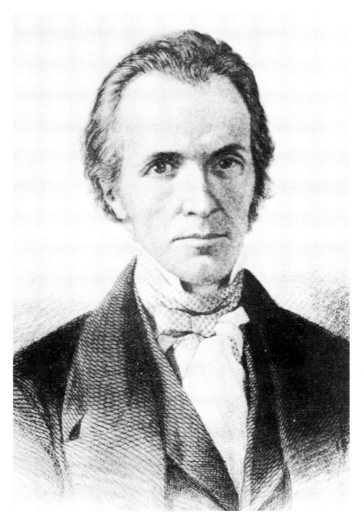

FIG. 3. Amariah Brigham. (From ref. 16.)

legally changed his name to Brown-Séquard. He received his medical education in Paris, where his doctoral thesis (1846) dealt with the reflex functions of the spinal cord. He was forced to leave France for political reasons in 1852, so he took a sailing boat for America, stating that he would learn English en route. He was unable to obtain an academic appointment and after a year he was allowed to return to France. In 1854, however, on the recommendation of his friend Paul Broca, he was appointed professor of the institutes of medicine (now the chair of physiology) at the Medical College of Virginia in Richmond. He was unhappy there—he was opposed to slavery,

AN INQUIRY

CONCERNING

THE DISEASES AND FUNCTIONS

OF

THE BRAIN,

THE SPINAL CORD,

AND

THE NERVES.

BY

AMARIAH BRIGHAM, M. D.

NEW-YORK.

GEORGE ADLARD, 168 BROADWAY

1840.

FIG. 4. Title page of Brigham's *An Inquiry Concerning the Diseases and Functions of the Brain, the Spinal Cord, and the Nerves.*

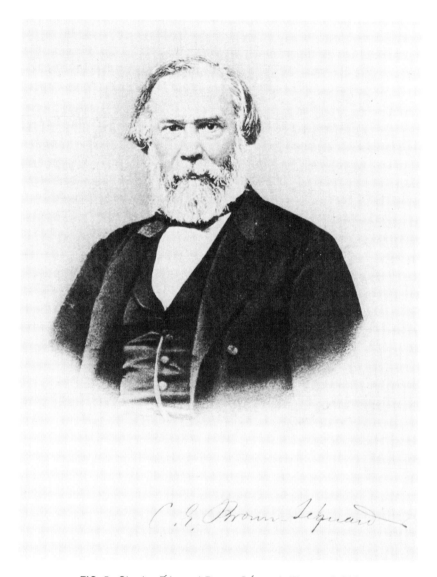

FIG. 5. Charles Édouard Brown-Séquard. (From ref. 22.)

he objected to the fact that he was expected to do didactic teaching rather than research, and his lectures were poorly received, in part because of his poor facility in English (29). He remained in Richmond only 3 or 4 months. In 1856–1857 Brown-Séquard gave a series of lectures on neurophysiologic topics in various American cities and several universities in Great Britain. In 1860 he was appointed one of the two original physicians to the National Hospital, Queen Square, London, where he remained for 4.5 years. In 1864 a new chair was established at Harvard Medical School, and Brown-Séquard was appointed professor of the physiology and pathology of the nervous system. Although he gave some highly appreciated lectures at Harvard, he was frequently absent on visits to Europe, and following the death of his first wife in 1867 he returned to Paris. In 1878, following the death of Claude Bernard, Brown-Séquard was appointed professor of experimental physiology at the College de France, where he remained until his death in 1894. During the later years of his life Brown-Séquard's principal research interests were in the field of endocrinology.

Brown-Séquard was an outstanding neurophysiologist, and his observations were important to an understanding of the functions of the nervous system. His *Course of Lectures on the Physiology and Pathology of the Central Nervous System,* published in 1860 (4), were lectures that had been delivered before the Royal College of Surgeons of London in May 1858. His contributions to clinical neurology, however, were not significant. Although he made many visits to the United States, he held only brief academic appointments there. He actually played an insignificant role in the development of American neurology.

REFERENCES

1. Bell, C. (1830): *The Nervous System of the Human Body.* Longmans, London.
2. Binger, C. A. L. (1966): *Revolutionary Doctor: Benjamin Rush.* Norton, New York.
3. Brigham, A. (1849): *An Inquiry Concerning the Diseases and Functions of the Brain, Spinal Cord, and Nerves.* George Adkard, New York.
4. Brown-Séquard, C. E. (1860): *Course of Lectures on the Physiology and Pathology of the Central Nervous System.* Collins, Philadelphia.
5. Cooke, J. A. (1820): *A Treatise on Nervous Disease.* Longmans, London.
6. Critchley, M. (1960): The beginnings of the National Hospital: Queen Square (1859–1860). *Br. Med. J.,* 1:1829–1831.
7. DeJong, R. N. (1940): The first American textbook on psychiatry: A review and discussion of Benjamin Rush's "Medical Inquiries and Observations upon the Diseases of the Mind." *Ann. Med. Hist.,* 2:195–202. (3rd series).
8. Dunglison, R. (1842): *The Practice of Medicine, or, A Treatise in Special Pathology and Therapeutics.* Lae and Blanchard, Philadelphia.
9. Farr, C. B. (1944): Benjamin Rush and American psychiatry. *Am. J. Psychiatry,* 100:3–115.
10. Flexner, J. T. (1937): *Doctors on Horseback: Pioneers of American Medicine.* Viking Press, New York.
11. Garrison, F. H. (1929): *An Introduction to the History of Medicine,* 4th Ed. Saunders, Philadelphia.
12. Hall, M. (1836): *Lectures on the Nervous System and Its Diseases.* Sherwood, Gilbert and Piper, London.
13. Hammond, W. A. (1883): *A Treatise on Insanity in Its Medical Relations.* Appleton, New York.
14. Hammond, W. A. (1873): *Insanity in Its Relation to Crime.* Appleton, New York.
15. Holmes, G. (1954): *The National Hospital Queen Square, 1860–1948.* Livingstone, Edinburgh and London.
16. Hutchings, R. H. (1944): Amariah Brigham: founder and first editor of the American Journal of Psychiatry. *Am. J. Psychiatry,* 100:29–33.
17. Jackson, J. (1855): *Letters to a Young Physician Just Entering Upon Practice.* Phillips, Simpson and Company, Boston.

18. Magendie, M. (1839): *Leçons sur les fonctions et maladies du systeme nerveux.* Libraire-Editeur, Chéz Ebrard.
19. Marshall, A. (1815): *The Morbid Anatomy of the Brain in Mania and Hydrophobia with the Pathology of These Two Diseases.* Longman, Hurst, Rees, Orme, and Brown, London.
20. McHenry, L. C., Jr. (1969): *Garrison's History of Neurology.* Charles C Thomas, Springfield, Illinois.
21. Mills, C. K. (1886–1887): Benjamin Rush and American psychiatry. *Medico-legal J.,* 4:238–273.
22. Olmsted, J. M. D. (1946): *Charles-Édouard Brown-Séquard: A Nineteenth Century Neurologist and Endocrinologist.* Johns Hopkins Press, Baltimore.
23. Olmsted, J. M. D. (1970): Édouard Brown-Séquard (1871–1894). In: *The Founders of Neurology,* 2nd Ed, edited by W. Haymaker and F. Schiller., pp. 181–186. Charles C Thomas, Springfield, Illinois.
24. Pepper, W. (1890): Benjamin Rush. *J.A.M.A.* 14:593–595.
25. Romberg, M. H. (1853): *A Manual of the Nervous Diseases of Man.,* translated by E. H. Sieveking. The Sydenham Society, London.
26. Rush, B. (1812): *Medical Inquiries of Observations Upon the Diseases of the Mind.* Kimber & Richardson, Philadelphia.
27. Shyrock, R. H. (1971): The medical reputation of Benjamin Rush. *Bull. Hist. Med.,* 45:507–515.
28. Spitzka, E. C. (1883): *Insanity, Its Classificaion, Diagnosis and Treatment: A Manual for Students and Practitioners of Medicine.* Bermingham & Co., New York.
29. Tucker, W. M. (1973): The history of neurology in the state of Virginia (1854–1973). *Va. Med. Mon.,* 100:927–929.

2

The Beginnings
of American Neurology

Silas Weir Mitchell and William Alexander Hammond have been called the fathers of American neurology. They specialized in the diagnosis and treatment of diseases of the nervous system and were authors of the first, and some of the most important, treatises on neurologic disease. They were also the pioneer American neurologic investigators.

Silas Weir Mitchell (1829–1914) (Fig. 6) came from a family of wealth and culture in early Philadelphia (3,8,18,53,54). He was a son and grandson of physicians and, in fact, was the seventh physician in three generations of his family. His father was John Kearsley Mitchell, who for many years was professor of the practice of medicine at the Jefferson Medical College. Mitchell was not only an erudite and versatile neurologist, he was also a physiologist, psychiatrist, novelist, and poet. He was elected president of the American Neurological Association when it was founded in 1875, but because he was not able to attend the first meeting he asked that his name be withdrawn from the list of officers. He did serve as president of the Association in 1909, however, 5 years before his death.

Mitchell entered the University of Pennsylvania at the age of 15, but did poorly as a student because of his widespread interests. When he decided to go into medicine his father told him, "You have no appreciation of the life [of a doctor]. You are wanting in nearly all the qualities that go to make success in medicine. You have brains enough, but no industry" (3). In spite of this judgment, however, he entered Jefferson Medical College, from which he was graduated in 1850 at the age of 21, following which he went to Europe where he worked with Pierre Robin and Claude Bernard. He was greatly influenced by Bernard, who stimulated his interest in research. When discussing a certain hypothesis with the great physiologist, he stated that "I think that so and so must be the case." Bernard's reply, which left a deep impression on him, was, "Why think, when you can experiment? Exhaust experiment and then think" (3).

On returning to Philadelphia, Mitchell entered private practice with his

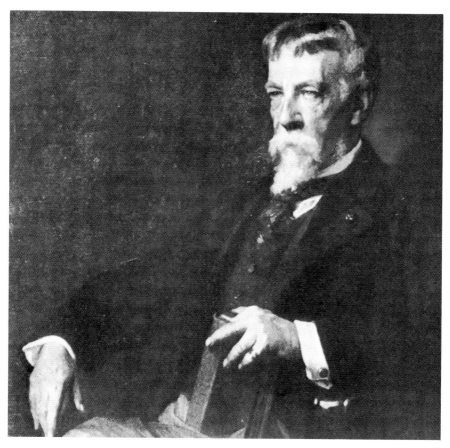

FIG. 6. S. Weir Mitchell. Vonnoh portrait, in the College of Physicians, Philadelphia. (From ref. 3).

father but also devoted a part of each day to research. He had become interested in microscopy from his work with Robin, and with his microscope he established a laboratory from which there emanated in rapid succession a number of reports, many of which were presented at meetings of the Philadelphia Academy of Natural Science and were published in its proceedings. They dealt with various subjects, mainly chemical and anatomic, but clinical reports were interspersed. Later studies were largely toxicologic ones, some dealing with snake venom and other toxins. Some of his investigations were carried out with collaborators, among them William A. Hammond, who was later to be Surgeon General of the United States Army. He published two papers jointly with Hammond (41,42). He worked long hours in the laboratory, often from three or four o'clock in the afternoon until one o'clock the next morning, and at the same time was building a busy practice.

When the Civil War broke out, Mitchell declined an appointment as brigade surgeon, feeling that he should remain at home and, for financial reasons, continue his practice: however, he did accept appointments for part-time duty in some of the army hospitals around Philadelphia. His first appointment was in the Filbert Street Hospital, and it was there that he "began to be interested in injuries and wounds of nerves, about which little was then known" (3). In consequence, other physicians who were not interested in patients with such problems began to arrange transfers to his ward. When Surgeon General Hammond established a small hospital for nervous diseases on Christian Street, Mitchell was appointed there. Another collaborator and a former classmate of Mitchell's, George R. Morehouse, became associated with him at the Christian Street Hospital. This facility soon became over-utilized, and Hammond established a new 400-bed hospital, the Turner's Lane Military Hospital. Mitchell and Morehouse transferred to the new facility, and William W. Keen was appointed assistant surgeon at Mitchell's request (25).

At this hospital the three investigators studied their patients in detail and made profuse notes regarding their clinical findings, although Mitchell and Morehouse continued with their private practices as well. They made early morning visits (at about 7 o'clock) to perform routine duties and then carried on with their practices, returning to the hospital at three or four o'clock and then, according to autobiographic notes, "worked on note-taking, often as late as twelve or one at night, and when we got through, walked home, talking over our cases. Usually the work took 4 or 5 hours and we did it all in person. The late hours came two or three times a week and usually followed an inflow of cases of injuries to nerves after some serious battle. I have worked with many men since, but never with men who took more delight to repay opportunity with labor . . . the opportunity was indeed unique, and we knew it. The cases were of amazing interest. Here at the time were 80 epileptics and every kind of nerve wound, palsies, choreas, stump disorders. I sometimes wondered how we stood it" (3). These investigations resulted in the publication of a series of well-known papers and one book which revolutionized knowledge of nerve injuries, *Gunshot Wounds and Other Injuries of Nerves* (45). Mitchell published a more extensive study in 1872, *Injuries of Nerves and Their Consequences* (30). On the dedication page of this book Mitchell stated "To Wm. A. Hammond, M.D., Professor of Diseases of the Mind and Nervous System and of Clinical Medicine in the Bellevue Hospital Medical College, New York, whose life and views created the special hospital which furnished the chief experiences of this volume; with admiration for his high qualities as physician and scholar, and with grateful memories of a long and constant friendship, I dedicate the following pages." In the preface he stated that he was largely indebted for the assistance of Drs. George Morehouse and W. W. Keen, his former colleagues at the U.S.A. Hospital for Injuries and Diseases of the Nervous System. This book was to be the standard reference work on nerve injuries until the First World War. It went through many editions and was translated into several languages. Mitchell's son, John Kearsly Mitchell, completed the trilogy with a follow-up of many of the original cases, *Remote Consequences of Injuries of Nerves and Their Treatment* (29).

In addition to the descriptions of the characteristic motor and sensory deficits observed following injuries to peripheral nerves, Mitchell introduced the term "causalgia" for the dramatic complex of agonizing, burning pain, hypesthesia, and peripheral autonomic nervous system manifestations seen in some peripheral nerve injuries. His vivid description of the disorder has not been improved on. Apparently there was some skepticism about the syndrome on the part of Mitchell's contemporaries, who believed that the patients must have been exaggerating their symptoms. Mitchell replied to this by stating: "An English writer declares that he has never seen causalgia such as we saw from 1861 to 1864, nor have I seen it since, because men worn out with marching, soaked with malaria, and exhausted by exposure and diarrhea are not now the subjects of wounds from mini-balls" (33). Other aspects of injury to, and diseases of, the peripheral nervous system were also described by Mitchell, including phantom pain, disorders of stumps, the relationship between barometric pressure and neuralgia, regeneration after nerve section, postparalytic chorea, and erythromelalgia.

Reflex paralysis was the subject of a brief publication by Mitchell, Morehouse, and Keen in 1864 (46). They noted that on rare occasions they had encountered cases "in which paralysis of a remote part or parts has been occasioned by a gunshot wound of some prominent nerve or of some part of the body which is richly supplied by nerve branches of secondary size and importance." They reported only seven instances of such paralysis. The concept was only theoretical at best and could not be explained in neurophysiologic terms or verified neuropathologically. Some critics have expressed the opinion that they were describing contralateral paralysis with lesions of the motor cortex of the brain, anticipating the work of Fritsch and Hitzig, which was to be announced 5 years later. Seventy-seven years later the Yale University Medical School republished the article as an example of brilliant pioneering in medical research. In an introduction John F. Fulton stated: "The book on gunshot wounds and the circular which preceded it thus stand as one of the great milestones in the history of American neurology and American clinical medicine" (10). One wonders, however, if this interpretation of so-called reflex paralysis is correct. In 4 of the 7 reported cases the injury was to the thigh, in one to the neck, in one to the deltoid, and in one to the testicle. In most cases there was no loss of consciousness, and in none was there evidence of cerebral involvement. Recovery in most was spontaneous and complete, and in some it followed "faradization" (10). The paralysis in these cases was probably not organic in origin. The concept of reflex paralysis has no neurophysiologic basis, and the publication of the circular was unfortunate.

After the war Mitchell resumed the practice of general medicine. Over the next several years, however, his interest in injuries and diseases of the nerves became better known, and there was a gradual change in his practice. He stated, in his autobiographic notes, "Shortly after the war I began to find that, in consequence of my published papers, I was being consulted more and more about nervous maladies. This intruded on my morning hours, so that my new work interfered with my private practice. This had been extremely large. [It grew to be at one time probably the largest in Philadelphia.] I found, however, that my income was not injured by the change. It ended in a few years by my dropping out of general practice and becoming principally a consultant in the nervous diseases. A book that I wrote during the war on 'Injuries and Diseases of Nerves' contributed to increase this special form of work" (3). He had increasing numbers of referrals of patients with diagnostic problems, many of them labeled hysterical. These cases are described in his books *Clinical Lectures on Nervous Diseases* (31) and *Lectures on Diseases of the Nervous System, Especially in Women;* the latter was dedicated "to J. Hughlings Jackson, M.D., F.R.S., with warm personal regards, and in grateful acknowledgement of his services to the science of medicine" (32). He continued, however, with his research, doing studies of nerve irritation and on the physiology of the cerebellum (33). In the latter studies he worked mainly with birds, and he referred frequently to the investigations carried out by Magendie. Mitchell supported the view that the cerebellum augments and reinforces movement. He was among the first to test the tendon reflexes as a part of the neurologic examination, and with Lewis (1886) showed that they can be reinforced by sensory stimuli (43,44). He also conducted experimental studies on the cremasteric reflex (34).

In 1871 Mitchell published *Wear and Tear,* the first of his series of books on medical matters addressed primarily to the laity (35). The theme of the book was a concern over increasing urban pressures and their effect on American life, resulting in an increase of "nervous diseases." "*Wear* is a natural and legitimate result of lawful use, and what we all have to put up with. Long strain, or the sudden demand of strength from weakness, causes *tear*. Wear comes of use, tear of abuse." This was followed by *Nurse and Patient and Camp Cure* (36), and later by *Fat and Blood—and How to Make Them* (37). These books were highly popular, and many editions were published. The choice of the title of *Fat and Blood* was somewhat unfortunate, and in later editions a subtitle was added which was more descriptive of the book: *An Essay on the Treatment of Certain Forms of Neurasthenia and Hysteria.* It was on the basis of these books and other of Mitchell's writings that the concept of his well-known "rest cure" was developed (38,39). This consisted of an elaborate and individualized use of initial isolation of the patient, insistence on prolonged bed rest and professional nursing, extensive concern about nutrition and the use of a high-calorie diet, the utilization of massage and other forms of physiotherapy, and "moral therapy." Each of these had been used in the past, but never in combination. This regimen was rigidly followed by many physicians over a considerable period of time.

Most of Mitchell's career, in addition to an extremely large private practice, was spent in clinical work at the Orthopaedic Hospital and Infirmary for Nervous Diseases, where there were outpatient and inpatient services for neurologic patients (Fig. 7). His many papers show his preoccupation with treatment in neurology. In his talks before local and national medical societies, he repeatedly called for greater attention to methods of treatment and found this subject lacking in most scientific programs.

To Mitchell's deep regret, he was never offered a professorship. On more than one occasion he was considered seriously for the chair of physiology at Jefferson Medical College and the University of Pennsylvania, but on each occasion the position was offered to someone else. He personally thought that there were political reasons for this, and he was probably correct. He

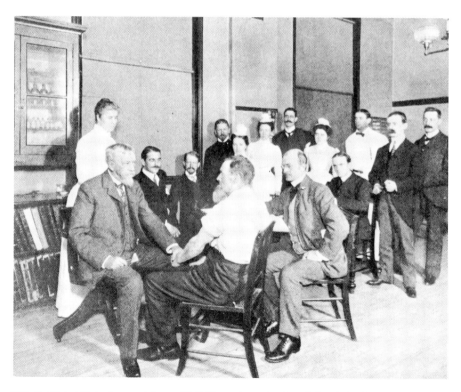

FIG. 7. Weir Mitchell examining a Civil War veteran in the clinic of the Orthopaedic Hospital and Infirmary for Nervous Diseases. (From ref. 3.)

played very active roles, however, in the Philadelphia Neurological Society and the Philadelphia College of Physicians, and had personal contacts with and greatly influenced the careers of many Philadelphia neurologists and neurosurgeons, including Charles K. Mills, Wharton Sinkler, William G. Spiller, Charles W. Burr, and his own son John K. Mitchell. He also influenced the careers of others, including Sir William Osler and Hideyo Noguchi. One of his pupils, Mills, was appointed the first professor of neurology at the University of Pennsylvania in 1903.

In 1894 Mitchell, who certainly practiced psychiatry as well as neurology but called himself a neurologist, was asked to address the semicentennial meeting of the American Medico-Psychological Association (now the American Psychiatric Association) (40). While preparing for this lecture he sought information about psychiatry and psychiatric "asylums" from such outstanding physicians as Billings, Dana, Hammond, Jacobi, Lyman, Mills, Osler, Putnam, and Sinkler. At the meeting he gave an address which was highly critical of existing institutions and psychiatric practice. He chided the psychiatrists for their isolation. "Once we spoke of asylums with respect, it is not so now. We neurologists think you have fallen behind us, and this opinion is gaining ground outside our ranks, and is, in part at least, your own fault. Where are your careful scientific reports? You live alone, uncriticized, unquestioned, out of the healthy conflicts and honest rivalries which keep us [neurologists] up to the mark of the fullest possible competence." This criticism, in part at least, led to much controversy and very likely had a favorable influence on later psychiatric research.

In addition to his career as a neurologist, physician, and investigator, Mitchell achieved considerable fame as an author and poet. He wrote some poems during his college years, his first published poem, "To a Polar Star," appearing in the *Nassau Monthly* in 1846. His first short story, "The Case of George Dedlow" (actually a case report), was submitted to the *Atlantic Monthly* without his knowledge and was published anonymously in 1866, and in 1867 "The Autobiography of a Quack" was published serially in the same magazine. In an 1864 letter to his sister Elizabeth he stated, "It occurred to me to see if I could write a story in my idle hours" (3). His first signed novel was *In War Time*, published in 1884, and his second novel, *Roland Blake*, appeared in 1886. In all he published 19 novels, seven books of poetry, short stories, children's stories, and a scholarly but controversial life of George Washington. His "Ode on a Lycian Tomb" has been said to be the finest elegaic poem written in America, and *Hugh Wynne, Free Quaker* was one of the most popular novels of its time. His novels were successful in part because of their detailed character delineation, made possible for the most part as a result of Mitchell's great clinical experience, particularly with hysteria. Throughout his literary career he utilized the experiences he had had in his medical research and practice. His characters were often based on neurologic and psychiatric patients he had come to know. In a letter used as a preface to Rein's book *S. Weir Mitchell as a Psychiatric Novelist,* he is quoted as saying, "I find, always, a little to my surprise, sometimes to my regret, that I get a clinical picture into my books of some form of mental disorder. When somebody, if ever, comes to review my books as a whole, he will probably recognize with astonishment that they include a clinical study of various forms of psychic disorder" (50). Characters in his books include alcoholics with varying degrees of affliction, "couch-loving invalids" reminiscent of Victorian hypochondriacs, those with dual personalities, persons with intellectual and character deterioration, and a few psychotics. Several doctors are included in the characters he described, but none was autobiographical. In spite of his literary success, when asked near the end of his life, "Would you rather be remembered for your literary work or your medical work?" he promptly replied "Medical, of course" (3).

Although he never held an academic appointment, Mitchell was awarded honorary degrees by many universities, including Bologna, Edinburgh, Harvard, Johns Hopkins, Princeton, and Toronto; and for many years he served on the Board of Trustees of the University of Pennsylvania. He was a striking and distinguished person, with a rich background of general culture. He was energetic and self-confident, and with friends and patients he had charm, sympathy, and patience. He was outgoing and had many friends with whom he actively corresponded, including Charles Francis Adams, Louis Agassiz, John Shaw Billings, Phillips Brooks, Andrew Carnegie, Ralph Waldo Emerson, Simon Flexner, John Hay, Oliver Wendell Holmes, Henry and William James, James Russell Lowell, George Meredith, Charles Elliot Norton, Sir William Osler, Francis Parkman, James Whitcomb Riley, Sir Ronald Ross, Augustus and Homer St. Gaudens, John Singer Sargeant, Alfred Lord Tennyson, Walt Whitman, William Welch, and Owen Wister. He continued to be active in practice, productive in literature, and vigorous until his death at the age of 84.

A contemporary, close friend, and one-time collaborator of Mitchell's was **William Alexander Hammond** (1828–1900) (Fig. 8) (19,20,22). Born in Annapolis, Maryland, the son of a physician, Hammond studied medicine at New York University from which he graduated in 1848. After a brief period at the Pennsylvania Hospital, he enlisted in the United States Army as an assistant surgeon and served at various posts in New Mexico, Kansas, and Florida, as well as at West Point. He participated in many Indian campaigns, and he occupied his leisure time with physiologic and botanical studies. By 1860, however, he had become interested in academic affairs and resigned from the army to accept the appointment as professor of anatomy and physiology at the University of Maryland.

At the outbreak of the Civil War he re-entered the army and, having lost his seniority, was again made an assistant surgeon. Because of his previous military experience, he was assigned to administrative work in the organization of hospitals and sanitary stations. His accomplishments as medical in-

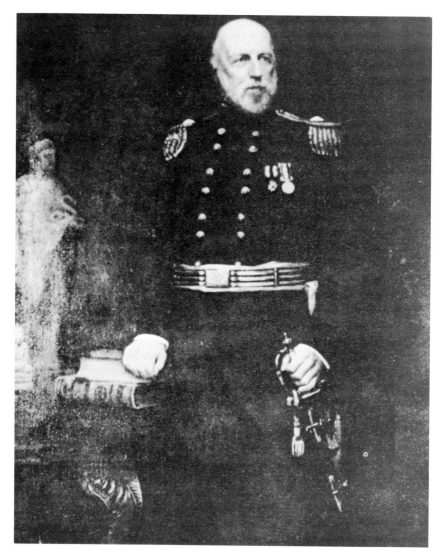

FIG. 8. William A. Hammond. Portrait in the National Library of Medicine. (From ref. 19.)

spector of camps and hospitals was said to be so outstanding that, at the urging of the Sanitary Commission and the advice of General McClellan, President Lincoln appointed him Surgeon General of the United States Army in 1862 at the age of 34. The work of the Surgeon General's office at once assumed an aspect of efficiency and force, but the promotion of Hammond over the heads of the Assistant Surgeon General and the rest of the staff did not fail to arouse antagonism among his colleagues. His forceful administration clashed most particularly with the autocratic spirit of Edmund M. Stanton, Secretary of War, and this came to a climax when Hammond was ordered on an extended, presumably permanent, inspection tour. Hammond then requested either restoration of all of the prerogatives of office or trial by court martial. The latter was ordered, and he was tried in 1864 on the charge of irregularities in the purchase of medical supplies. A verdict of guilty was returned, and he was dismissed from the Army. This decision was later (1878) found to be unjust, however, and was reversed by Congress. He was then placed on the retired list with the full rank of Brigadier General, which he had previously held.

During his brief period of service as Surgeon General (April 28, 1862 to August 18, 1864) Hammond accomplished many reforms in army medical administration and made numerous important contributions. He founded the Army Medical Museum, since 1949 called the Armed Forces Institute of Pathology. He inaugurated and began compiling the *Medical and Surgical History of the War of the Rebellion*. He introduced the pavilion system of hospital construction throughout the service, as well as the development of specialty hospitals, such as the Turner's Lane Hospital where Mitchell did his significant work. He saw to it that there was a liberal supply of medical books and journals for the officers of the department, which greatly contributed to maintaining the army's high standards of medical practice. Many other reforms which later became realities were also recommended by him, including the formation of a permanent hospital corps, the establishment of an army medical school, the location of a permanent army general hospital in Washington, D.C., and the establishment of a military medical laboratory.

After his dismissal from the army, Hammond went to New York City where he entered the practice of neurology and psychiatry and made many important contributions to these fields. He was appointed lecturer in neurology and psychiatry at the College of Physicians and Surgeons in 1874 and professor of nervous and mental diseases at the Bellevue Hospital Medical College in 1876. He also taught at New York University and was one of the founders of the New York Postgraduate Medical School.

In 1871 Hammond published the first edition of his book *A Treatise on Diseases of the Nervous System* (11), the first American textbook of neurology. It went through seven editions within 10 years and was translated into several languages. In 1873 he published *Insanity in Its Relations to Crime* (12) and in 1874 *Clinical Lectures on Diseases of the Nervous System* (13). These are only three of the many books by him on nervous and mental diseases (14–16). His text *A Treatise on Insanity in Its Medical Relations* appeared in 1883 (17). From 1867 to 1872 he edited the *Quarterly Journal of Physiological Medicine and Medical Jurisprudence,* from 1867 to 1879 he was editor of the *New York Medical Journal,* and between 1879 and 1881 he and William G. Morton published three issues of *Neurological Contributions.*

Hammond conducted many original investigations and described several hitherto unrecorded conditions. His best known contribution to the description of neurologic symptomatology is his delineation of the condition now known as athetosis (without fixed position), although in the beginning Mitchell called it hemichorea and Gowers termed it mobile spasm. He stated that the probable seat of the morbid process was in the corpus striatum, and postmortem examination of one of his patients 20 years later proved him correct. As a teacher he aroused the enthusiastic interest of students and was most effective in convincing the medical profession of the importance of the neurologic sciences.

Hammond was tall and commanding in appearance, and had a powerful voice. He was an outstanding leader and talented organizer. He was one of the founders of the American Neurological Association, of which he was president in 1882. The invitations to attend the organizing meeting were sent out from his office, and he played an important role in the Association's early success.

Like Mitchell, Hammond also had literary interests, and he wrote novels and plays. Also like Mitchell, he had a son who became a neurologist, Graeme Monroe Hammond (who incidentally was president of the American Neurological Association in 1899). Hammond shares with Mitchell the distinction of having secured for neurology its place in the orbit of American medicine. In 1878 he returned to Washington, D.C., where he became interested in the subject of animal extracts and was largely instrumental in their introduction into clinical use. He lived in Washington until his death in 1900.

During and immediately after the pioneering work of Mitchell and Hammond, the specialty of neurology developed spontaneously in medical centers throughout the United States. This took place most frequently in the large cities in the eastern seaboard, where the centers of population were located, but also farther west in such cities as Cincinnati and Chicago, and even as far west as St. Louis and New Orleans. It was to appear later west of the Mississippi, but migration into the western states was just beginning at the time of the Civil War. The physicians who did early work on diseases of the nervous system, however, did not call themselves neurologists. Some were internists or practitioners of general medicine who happened to have a special interest in diseases of the nervous system. Many, like Mitchell and Hammond, were interested in diseases of the mind as well as of the nervous system. Some, fascinated by the recent work of Duchenne and Erb, who electrically stimulated muscles and nerves, became interested in diseases of the nervous system following the advent of electrodiagnosis and so-called electrotherapy.

An early Baltimore neurologist was **Francis Turquand Miles** (1827–1903) (23,52). He was born near Charleston, South Carolina, and received his medical degree from the Medical College of South Carolina in

1849. He studied in France under Charcot and returned to the Medical College of South Carolina where he was first assistant demonstrator of anatomy and then professor of physiologic anatomy. At the outbreak of the Civil War, Miles joined the Confederate Army, where he rose to the rank of captain. He was discharged from the army after receiving several wounds and then joined its medical department. At the close of the war he returned to his faculty appointment but soon went to Europe for further study, this time in London. There he met and became friends with Jackson and Gowers. He returned to Charleston but in 1868 moved to Baltimore to join others who had served in the Confederate Army in organizing the Washington University School of Medicine. In 1869 Washington University was merged with the University of Maryland, and Miles joined that faculty as clinical professor of diseases of the nervous system and professor of general, descriptive, and surgical anatomy. In 1880 he abandoned anatomy to become professor of physiology, and he carried two titles—in neurology and physiology—until his retirement in 1903. He was the author of many papers and case reports, most of which were published in the now defunct *Baltimore Medical Journal,* and he contributed articles to several medical encyclopedias. He was one of the charter members of the American Neurological Association in 1880 and served as its second president.

Roberts Bartholow (1831–1904) was the third president of the American Neurological Association, serving in this position in 1881 (23). He was born in New Windsor, Maryland, and obtained his medical degree from the University of Maryland in 1852. He served as an army surgeon in the western frontier states and then had 3 years of military surgical experience during the Civil War. After the war he established a medical practice in Cincinnati and was appointed professor of materia medica and therapeutics and of the practice of medicine in the Medical College of Ohio in Cincinnati. He was a highly skilled practitioner and teacher but also carried out important and daring clinical investigations. In 1874 he decided to confirm in the human the work that Fritsch, Hitzig, and Ferrier had carried out on motor localization in the brains of experimental animals. He became the first to stimulate electrically the brain of a conscious human being. Mary Rafferty, a 30-year-old mentally retarded servant girl, dying with a rapidly expanding, malignant epithelioma, consented to his investigations. Hairless since a fall into a fire during infancy, she developed a small ulcer on her scalp, supposedly produced by friction from a piece of whalebone in her wig (2). This expanded, and when Bartholow saw her she had large open, purulent lesions over both parietal areas, with exposure of the dura mater. He inserted wires through the dura and into the brain and stimulated first one side and then the other with a faradic current. Muscular contractions occurred in the contralateral extremities, and on increasing the current a focal clonic convulsion took place. She died some days later following extension of the neoplasm with thrombosis of the superior longitudinal sinus. Bartholow was severely criticized at home and abroad for this investigation but defended himself admirably. In 1879 he moved to Philadelphia to accept the chair of materia medica and therapeutics at the Jefferson Medical College. His *Materia Medica and Therapeutics* was published in 1876. *A Treatise on the Practice of Medicine,* first published in 1880, went through 11 editions and was translated into Japanese. He retired from teaching and was made emeritus professor in 1903. He died in Philadelphia in 1904.

James Steward Jewell (1837–1887) was the most widely influential and scholarly pioneer in neurology in the Middle West (Fig. 9) (24). Born of poor parents near Galena, Illinois, he was the oldest of eight children. During early life he showed a love of learning and at the age of 18 began the study of medicine under the preceptorship of Dr. S. M. Mitchell of Corinth, Illinois.

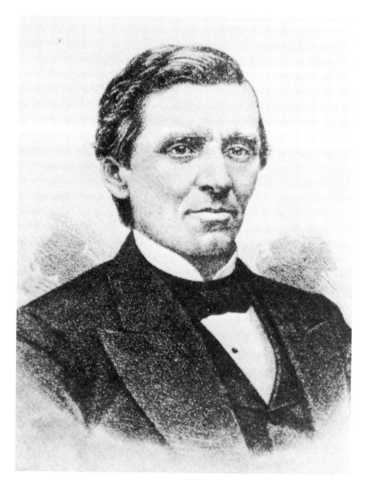

FIG. 9. James S. Jewell. (From ref. 24.)

In 1858 he went to Chicago to continue his medical education at Rush Medical College and later at the Medical Department of Lund University, from which he received his medical degree in 1860. Even before graduation he began teaching anatomy, and after graduation he entered the practice of general medicine, at the same time studying intensely and acquiring a good reading knowledge of French, German, and Italian and wide knowledge of Greek and Latin. In 1862 he was appointed professor of anatomy in the Chicago Medical College. He resigned from this position in 1869 at about the time that the institution became the medical department of Northwestern University. He then spent 2 years traveling in Europe and the Near East to study ancient and Biblical history for use in teaching a large Sunday School class in Evanston. On his return to Chicago in 1871, he resumed medical practice but restricted it to neurology and psychiatry with special emphasis on the former. In 1872 he was appointed professor of nervous and mental diseases at Northwestern University.

In 1874 Jewell and Henry M. Bannister founded and jointly edited the *Chicago Journal of Nervous and Mental Disease,* with Jewell as editor and Bannister as assistant editor. Two years later the word "Chicago" was dropped from the title of the journal, which has been published without interruption to the present time under the title of *Journal of Nervous and Mental Disease*. Jewell served as editor for 8 years. His editorial skills were exemplary and successful. He wrote the first article published in the journal, entitled "The Pathology of the Vasomotor Nervous System," and contributed many articles and editorials to subsequent issues. He was one of the seven signers of the original invitation to neurologists around the nation to meet in New York to form the American Neurological Association in 1875, and he served the Association as its president for its first 5 years. His health declined, and in 1884 he retired and moved to Florida, where he studied the cerebral anatomy of birds. After his return to Chicago in 1886 he founded a new journal, *The Neurological Review,* but his poor health forced him to suspend publication after only one volume had appeared. He died of pulmonary tuberculosis in 1887 at the age of 50.

Edward Constant Seguin (1843–1898) was born in Paris. He (Fig. 10) was the son of a physician, Edouard Seguin, who was known for his research on mental retardation (23). The elder Seguin moved his family to the United States in 1846, and his son studied at the College of Physicians and Surgeons in New York City, from which he graduated in 1864. In 1862 he was appointed a medical cadet in the Regular Army, and after his graduation he served as post surgeon in Little Rock, Arkansas, and at Fort Craig and Fort Selden in New Mexico. He spent the winter of 1869–1870 in Paris, studying under Brown-Séquard and Charcot, and became deeply interested in diseases of the nervous system. On his return to New York he was appointed professor of diseases of the nervous system at the College of Physicians and Surgeons, and he established a clinic for patients with these

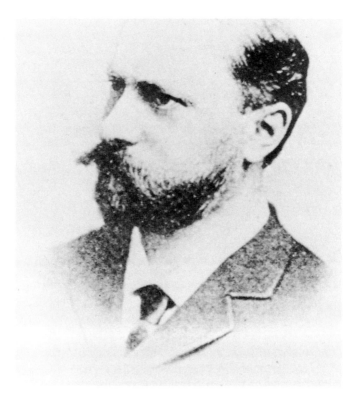

FIG. 10. Edward Constant Seguin. (From ref. 7a.)

diseases. Seguin's work as a teacher and writer was of the highest order. It was said that as a neurologic practitioner he would probably never be excelled. His contributions to the therapeutics of neurologic diseases were especially valuable. He wrote important papers on many neurologic subjects, and his lectures and papers on spastic paraplegia preceded those of Erb and Charcot. A series of papers on localization of brain lesions did a great deal to stimulate the study and practice of neurology in the United States. Seguin reported the first autopsied case of multiple sclerosis in the United States, a report that contained detailed histologic studies of the pons, medulla, and spinal cord, showing the early, more advanced and extensive manifestations of the disease. Although his chief interest was in diseases of the nervous system, it must not be forgotten that he played an important part in the introduction of medical thermometry in the United States. In collaboration with William H. Draper, professor of medicine in the College of Physicians and Surgeons, he devised the first clinical chart, showing in graphic form temperature, pulse, and respirations. He was a leader in the formation of the neurologic department of the Vanderbilt Clinic, a gift to the College of

Physicians and Surgeons in 1888 by the four sons of William K. Vanderbilt, and was the department's first director. The clinic served as an important training ground for neurologists and medical students until it closed in 1929 when the College of Physicians and Surgeons entered the Columbia-Presbyterian Medical Center.

He threw himself with great enthusiasm into literary ventures. In 1873 he joined with Brown-Séquard in the editorship of the *Archives of the Scientific Practice of Medicine,* a journal which did not, however, survive a year. Between 1876 and 1878 he edited a series of *American Clinical Lectures.* His most ambitious venture was the *Archives of Medicine,* in which an attempt was made to supply the profession with a superior journal. Founded in 1879, it was not a financial success, however, and publication ceased after the 12th volume. In 1884 he published a collection of his essays, articles, and lectures under the title *Opera Minora* (51). He also collaborated with his father in writing a book dealing with idiocy and its treatment. He was a founding member of the American Neurological Association and for several years was its secretary and treasurer, serving as its president in 1889. He spent several years abroad toward the end of his life. He resumed practice on his return to New York but did not resume his teaching. He died in 1898 at the age of 55.

James Jackson Putnam (1846–1918) was the son of a physician. His maternal grandfather, James Jackson, was the first physician to the Massachusetts General Hospital and a notable figure in early American medicine (7). Born in Boston, Putnam (Fig. 11) was graduated from Harvard Medical School in 1886, after which he served as house officer in Massachusetts General Hospital. He then went to Leipzig and Vienna where he worked with Rokitanksy and Meynert, and to London, where he was greatly impressed by Jackson. In 1872 he was appointed "electrician" to the Massachusetts General Hospital, and the following year his title was changed to physician to outpatients with diseases of the nervous system. In 1874 he was given the title lecturer on the application of electricity to nervous disease in the Harvard Medical School; 2 years later the title was changed to lecturer on diseases of the nervous system. In 1885 he was appointed instructor and in 1893 professor of diseases of the nervous system. He was particularly interested in physiology and pathology of the nervous system, which he studied with Henry P. Bowditch and William James. With the latter he experimented on the electrical stimulation of the cortex of the dog. Finding no facilities in either the hospital or the medical school for this work, he set up a laboratory in his own home where he carried out many of his early investigations.

In 1883 Putnam made a careful clinical and pathologic description of poliomyelitis. After this he investigated arsenical and lead neuropathies and beriberi. In 1890 he published the first of a series of papers dealing with what is now known as combined system disease. Although many of the patients were anemic and most had nutritional defects, the relationship of this syn-

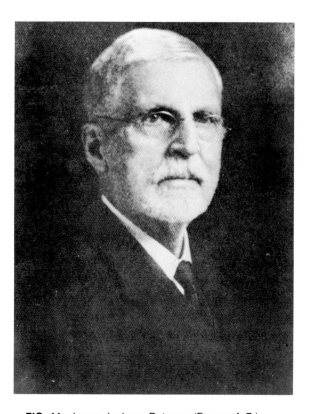

FIG. 11. James Jackson Putnam. (From ref. 7.)

drome to pernicious anemia was not recognized until later. Putnam was a founding member of the American Neurological Association and the Boston Society of Psychiatry and Neurology, and served as president of the former in 1888. He was interested, however, not only in organic diseases of the nervous system but also in the neuroses (49) and "neurasthenia." Between 1890 and 1910 he regularly attended meetings with philosophers and psychologists, e.g., William James, Josiah Royce, Hugo Munsterberg, Morton Prince, and Adolf Meyer, who was in Worcester, Massachusetts, from 1896 to 1902. He began to report on psychological studies more frequently (50). He became interested in psychoanalysis early in its development and was in part responsible for inducing Sigmund Freud to present his famous series of lectures at Clark University in Worcester in 1909. The lectures were followed by a visit by Freud and Jung to the Putnam-Bowditch summer camp at Keens Valley in the Adirondacks. Putnam's enthusiastic report on this visit to the American Neurological Association that year produced nine pages of debate. Putnam was appointed professor emeritus at Harvard Medical School in 1912, six years before his death.

Charles Karsner Mills (1845–1931) (Fig. 12) was born in Philadelphia. His early education was interrupted by the Civil War, during which he served in the Union Army (1,9). He was graduated from the medical department of the University of Pennsylvania in 1869 and received a Ph.D. degree from the same university in 1871. The university conferred the degree of LL.D. on him in 1916. At first Mills engaged in the practice of general medicine but soon became interested in nervous and mental diseases; within 10 years of starting practice, he was devoting his entire time to specializing in this branch of medicine. He was a great clinical neurologist and made many significant contributions to the specialty during its early growth. He had staff appointments at many Philadelphia hospitals, although his most important studies were on patients under his care at the Philadelphia General

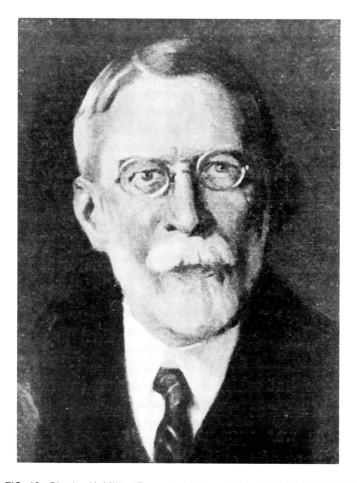

FIG. 12. Charles K. Mills. (From *Arch. Neurol. Psychiat.*, 26:171, 1931.)

Hospital, known familiarly in his time as "Old Blockley." He held teaching positions in many of the medical institutions in Philadelphia as well. He was professor of nervous and mental diseases in Philadelphia Polyclinic (1883–1898) and clinical professor of nervous diseases in the Women's Medical College of Pennsylvania (1891–1902). He served successively as lecturer on electrotherapeutics (1877), lecturer on nervous and mental diseases (1879), professor of mental disease and of medical jurisprudence (1893), and clinical professor of nervous diseases (1901) at the University of Pennsylvania, and was appointed professor of neurology there in 1903. This appointment was a significant one in that it indicated that his accomplishments had resulted in the establishment of neurology as an autonomous department in a major medical school. He was made professor emeritus in 1915.

Mills made many important contributions to neurology. In 1877 he established the neurology wards in the Philadelphia General Hospital with 20 beds for male and female patients. In 1878 there were 35 patients, and by 1910 the number of patients had reached 400. He did significant work on aphasia, cortical localization, and the symptomatology of parietal lobe and uncinate gyrus lesions (26). He was the first to describe geniculate neuralgia and macular hemianopia. In 1886, a year before Korsakoff's description in Russia, he described alcoholic polyneuropathy with psychic phenomena. In 1900 he described unilateral progressive ascending paralysis due to degeneration of the pyramidal tract, now known as Mills' syndrome (27). In 1912 he reported the first case of occlusion of the superior cerebellar artery.

Mills' textbook on neurology (28), published in 1898, admirably set forth his unusual clinical experience and received wide acclaim. In the preface he stated: "The great work of Gowers is the only extensive treatise on nervous diseases in the English language, although excellent manuals of moderate size have been written, and the author has been led to believe that a large textbook, including a comparatively full presentation of the many recent additions to the anatomy and pathology of the nervous system, would be in accord with the needs of the profession." The book, in contrast to that of Gowers, contains a lengthy section on the methods of examination of the nervous system and on the meaning of localizing signs, as well as numerous references to the anatomic literature. There is also an extensive bibliography. It is the first textbook on neurology to contain a section on the chemistry of the nervous system, with a reference to the work of Thudicum.

Mills was president of the American Neurological Association in 1886 and again in 1924 at the time of its semicentennial. In spite of his poor vision (for half of his life he was unable to read), he continued to be active and to contribute to the neurologic literature until the year of his death at the age of 86.

A man of this period who made a significant contribution to neurology even though he was not a neurologist was **George Sumner Huntington**

(1850–1916) (Fig. 13) (4–6,55). Huntington was born in East Hampton, New York, the son and grandson of physicians who had practiced there. He received his early clinical training from his father and then attended the College of Physicians and Surgeons of Columbia University, from which he graduated in 1871. He practiced briefly with his father, but later in 1871 he moved to Pomeroy, Ohio, to set up practice there. While still in East Hampton, however, he made preliminary notes for a paper on chorea and then wrote a preliminary draft of the paper. This was carefully reviewed by his father whose penciled notes and corrections can still be seen on the original manuscript. On February 15, 1872, less than a year after graduation from medical school, he read the paper before the Meiga and Mason

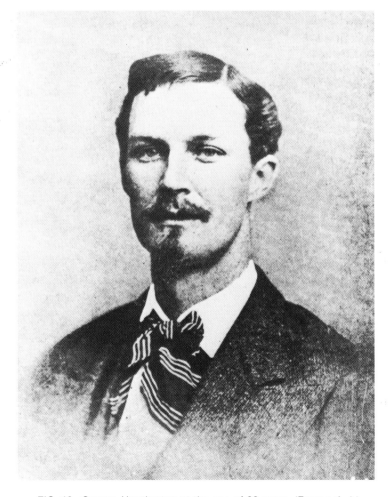

FIG. 13. George Huntington at the age of 22 years. (From ref. 4.)

Academy of Medicine in Middleport, Ohio, and because it was well received he sent it to the *Medical and Surgical Reporter* of Philadelphia, where it was published April 13, 1872 (21). In this report he described a hereditary form of chorea he had observed with his father on Long Island. It had its onset during adult life, had associated mental changes, was remorselessly progressive, and was transmitted from one generation to another. It has been known since as Huntington's chorea. There had been a few prior descriptions of the disease, but because of his concise and accurate account of the disorder it is appropriate that it bears Huntington's name. Sir William Osler, referring to Huntington's contribution, states: "In a postscript to an everyday sort of article on chorea minor he describes graphically in three or four paragraphs the characters of a chronic form which he, his father, and grandfather had observed in Long Island" (47). Later Osler wrote: "In the history of medicine there are few instances in which a disease has been more accurately, more graphically, or more briefly described" (48). Huntington was a family physician. He returned to New York State in 1874 and spent the rest of his active life in the practice of general medicine in Dutchess County until his retirement at the age of 65 years. He died the following year. His paper on chorea was his only contribution to the medical literature. Speaking before the New York Neurological Society in 1909, Huntington stated that without the facts and observations handed down to him by his grandfather and father, he could never have formulated a picture of the salient characteristics of the diseases so true and so complete as to make it a so-called classic (22).

REFERENCES

1. Alpers, B. J. (1975): Charles Karsner Mills (1845–1931). In: *Centennial Anniversary Volume of the American Neurological Association 1875–1975*, edited by D. Denny-Brown, A. S. Rose, and A. L. Sahs, pp. 80–84. Springer, New York.
2. Bartholow, R. (1874): Experimental investigations into the functions of the human brain. *Am. J. Med. Sci.*, 67:605–613.
3. Burr, A. R. (1929): *Weir Mitchell—His Life and Letters.* Duffield & Co., New York.
4. DeJong, R. N. (1937): George Huntington and his relationship to the earlier descriptions of chronic hereditary chorea. *Ann. Med. Hist.*, 9:201–210.
5. DeJong, R. N. (1970): George Huntington (1850–1916). In: *The Founders of Neurology*, 2nd Ed., edited by W. Haymaker and F. Schiller, pp. 453–456. Charles C Thomas, Springfield, Illinois.
6. DeJong, R. N. (1973): The history of Huntington's chorea in the United States. *Adv. Neurol.*, 1:19–27.
7. Denny-Brown, D. (1975): James Jackson Putnam (1845–1918). In: *Centennial Anniversary Volume of the American Neurological Association 1875–1975*, edited by D. Denny-Brown, A. S. Rose, and A. L. Sahs, pp. 86–90. Springer, New York.
7a. Denny-Brown, D., Rose, A. S., and Sahs, A. L., editors (1975): *Centennial Anniversary Volume of the American Neurological Association 1875–1975*, p. 92. Springer, New York.
8. Earnest, E. (1950): *S. Weir Mitchell: Novelist and Physician.* University of Pennsylvania Press, Philadelphia.
9. Frazier, C. H., Spiller, W. G., Burr, C. W., et al. (1932): Charles Karsner Mills: Memorial

Meeting of the Philadelphia Neurological Society. *Arch. Neurol. Psychiatry,* 28:1390–1410.

10. Fulton, J. F. (1941): *Introductory Note to Reflex Paralysis.* Historical Library, Yale University School of Medicine, New Haven.

11. Hammond, W. A. (1871): *A Treatise on Diseases of the Nervous System.* Appleton, New York.

12. Hammond, W. A. (1873): *Insanity in Its Relation to Crime.* Appleton, New York.

13. Hammond, W. A. (1874): *Clinical Lectures on Diseases of the Nervous System.* Appleton, New York.

14. Hammond, W. A. (1866): *On Wakefulness with an Introductory Chapter on Physiology of Sleep.* Lippincott, Philadelphia.

15. Hammond, W. A. (1878): *Cerebral Hypermia: The Result of Mental Strain or Emotional Disturbance.* Putnam, New York.

16. Hammond, W. A. (1881): *On Certain Conditions of Nervous Derangement: Somnambulism—Hypnotism—Hysteria—Hysteroid Affections, Etc.* Putnam, New York.

17. Hammond, W. A. (1883): *A Treatise on Insanity in Its Medical Relations.* Appleton, New York.

18. Haymaker, W. (1970): Wier Mitchell (1829–1914). In: *The Founders of Neurology,* 2nd Ed., edited by W. Haymaker and F. Schiller, pp. 479–484. Charles C Thomas, Springfield, Illinois.

19. Haymaker, W.: William Alexander Hammond (1828–1900). In: *The Founders of Neurology,* 2nd Ed., edited by W. Haymaker and F. Schiller, pp. 445–449. Charles C Thomas, Springfield, Illinois.

20. Heck, A. F. (1963): William Alexander Hammond—1828–1900. *J.A.M.A., 183:466–468.*

21. Huntington, G. (1872): On chorea. *Med. Surg. Rep., 24:317–321.*

22. Huntington, G. (1910): Recollections of Huntington's chorea as I saw it at East Hampton, Long Island, during my boyhood. *J. Nerv. Ment. Dis., 37:255–257.*

23. Kelly, H. A., and Burrage, W. L. (1920): *American Medical Biographies.* Norman Remington Company, Baltimore.

24. Mackay, R. P. (1975): James Stewart Jewell (1837–1887). In: *Centennial Anniversary Volume of the American Neurological Association 1875–1975,* edited by D. Denny-Brown, A. S. Rose, and A. L. Sahs. pp. 64–67. Springer, New York.

25. Middleton, W. S. (1966): Turner's Lane Hospital. *Bull. Hist. Med., 40:14–42.*

26. Mills, C. K. (1904): Aphasia and the cerebral zone of speech. *Am. J. Med. Sci., 128:375–393.*

27. Mills, C. K. (1900): A case of unilateral ascending paralysis. *J. Nerv. Ment. Dis., 27:195–200.*

28. Mills, C. K. (1898): *The Nervous System and Its Diseases: A Practical Treatise on Neurology for the Use of Physicians and Students.* Lippincott, Philadelphia.

29. Mitchell, J. K. (1895): *Remote Consequences of Injuries of Nerves and Their Treatment.* Lea Brothers, Philadelphia.

30. Mitchell, S. W. (1972): *Injuries of Nerves and Their Consequences.* Lippincott, Philadelphia.

31. Mitchell, S. W. (1897): *Clinical Lectures on Nervous Diseases.* Lea Brothers, Philadelphia.

32. Mitchell, S. W. (1881): *Lectures on Diseases of the Nervous System, Especially in Women.* Henry C. Lea's Sons & Co., Philadelphia.

33. Mitchell, S. W. (1869): Researches on the physiology of the cerebellum. *Am. J. Med. Sci., 37:320–338.*

34. Mitchell, S. W. (1879): The cremaster reflex. *J. Nerv. Ment. Dis. 6:577–586.*

35. Mitchell, S. W. (1871): *Wear and Tear.* Lippincott, Philadelphia.

36. Mitchell, S. W. (1877): *Nurse and Patient and Camp Cure.* Lippincott, Philadelphia.

37. Mitchell, S. W. (1877): *Fat and Blood—and How to Make Them.* Lippincott, Philadelphia.

38. Mitchell, S. W. (1875): Rest in nervous disease: its use and abuse. In: *A Series of American Clinical Lectures,* Vol 1, edited by E. C. Seguin, pp. 83–102.

39. Mitchell, S. W.: The treatment by rest, isolation, seclusion, etc. in relation to psychotherapy. *J.A.M.A., 50:2033–2037.*

40. Mitchell, S.W. (1894): Address before the fiftieth annual meeting of the American Medico-Psychological Association: Philadelphia, May 16th, 1894. *J. Nerv. Ment. Dis., 21:413–437.*

41. Mitchell, S. W., and Hammond, W. A. (1859): Experimental study of toxicological effects of sassy bark, the ordeal poison of the western coast of Africa. *Charleston Med. J.,* 14:721–740.
42. Mitchell, S. W., and Hammond, W. A. (1859): Experimental researches relative to corroval and vao—two new varieties of woorara, the South American arrow poison. *Am. J. Med. Sci.,* 38:13–60.
43. Mitchell, S. W., and Lewis, M. J. (1886): The tendon jerk and muscle jerk in disease, and especially in posterior sclerosis. *Am. J. Med. Sci.,* 93:363–372.
44. Mitchell, S. W., and Lewis, M. J. (1886): Physiological studies of the knee jerk, and of the reactions of muscles under mechanical and other excitants. *Med. News,* 48:169–173; 198–205.
45. Mitchell, S. W., Morehouse, G. R., and Keen, W. W. (1864): *Gunshot Wounds and Other Injuries of Nerves.* Lippincott, Philadelphia.
46. Mitchell, S. W., Morehouse, G. R., and Keen, W. W. (1964): *Reflex Paralysis.* Circular No. 6, Surgeon General's Office. March 10, 1964.
47. Osler, W. (1893): Remarks on the varieties of chronic chorea, and a report upon two families of the hereditary form, with one autopsy. *J. Nerv. Ment. Dis.,* 18:97–111.
48. Osler, W. (1908): Historical note on hereditary chorea. *Neurographs,* 1:113–116.
49. Putnam, J. J. (1910): On the etiology and treatment of the psychoneuroses. *Boston Med. Surg. J.,* 163:77–83.
50. Rein, D. (1952): *S. Weir Mitchell as a Psychiatric Novelist.* International Universities Press, New York.
51. Seguin, E. C. (1884): *Opera Minor: A Collection of Essays, Articles, Lectures, and Addresses.* Putnam, New York.
52. Van Buskirk, C. (1975): Francis Turquand Miles 1827–1903. In: *Centennial Anniversary Volume of the American Neurological Association, 1875–1975,* edited by D. Denny-Brown, A. S. Rose, and A. H. Sahs, pp. 68–69. Springer, New York.
53. Walter, R. D. (1970): *S. Weir Mitchell, M.D.—A Medical Biography.* Charles C Thomas, Springfield, Illinois.
54. Walter, R. D. (1975): Silas Weir Mitchell, 1829–1914. In: *Centennial Anniversary Volume of the American Neurological Association, 1875–1975,* edited by D. Denny-Brown, A. S. Rose, and A. L. Sahs. Springer, New York.
55. Whitfield, J. M. (1908): A biographical sketch of George Huntington, M.D. *Neurographs,* 1:89–93.

3

American Neurological Association

A critical and important development in American neurology took place in 1875 with the founding of the American Neurological Association (1,2). On December 15, 1874 the following letter was sent to physicians in various parts of the United States who were known to be especially interested in the diagnosis and treatment of diseases of the nervous system and in research in neurology:

Dear Sir:

It is contemplated to institute a society, to be called the American Neurological Association, to be devoted, as the name indicates, to the cultivation of Neurological Science in its normal and pathological relations. The number of members not to exceed fifty.

The Association will meet annually and continue its session several days. It is proposed to hold the first meeting in the city of New York, on Wednesday, the second day of June, 1875.

You are respectfully invited to participate in this meeting for organization, and to signify your acceptance or declination of this invitation to either of the undersigned at your earliest convenience.

Respectfully,
Your Obedient Servants,
William A. Hammond, M.D.
43 West 54th St., New York
Roberts Bartholow, M.D.
120 West 7th St., Cincinatti, Ohio
Meredith Clymer, M.D.
65 West 38th St., New York
J. S. Jewell, M.D.
57 Washington St., Chicago, Illinois
E. C. Seguin, M.D.
17 East 21st St., New York
James J. Putnam, M.D.
6 Park Square, Boston
T. M. B. Cross, M.D.
37 West 21st St., New York

This communication, sponsored as it was by men of distinction in several cities, received a warm response, and the following 28 physicians sent letters of acceptance: S. Weir Mitchell, Philadephia; J. K. Bauduy, St. Louis; F. D. Lente, Cold Spring, N.Y.; J. J. Mason, New York; John C. Shaw, Brooklyn; F. P. Kinnicutt, New York; A. D. Rockwell, New York; D. St. John Roosa, New York; A. McLane Hamilton, New York; S. G. Webber, Boston; D. F. Lincoln, Boston; E. C. Loring, New York; J. C. Dalton, New York; E. R. Hun, Albany, N.Y.; E. H. Clarke, Boston; H. D. Schmidt, New Orleans; S. M. Burnett, Knoxville, Tenn.; James Van Bibber, Baltimore; J. W. S. Arnold, New York; Robert T. Edes, Boston; N. B. Emerson, New York; T. A. McBride, New York; E. T. Miles, Baltimore; William Pepper, Philadelphia; H. C. Wood, Philadelphia; Walter Hay, Chicago; H. M. Bannister, Chicago; and J. S. Lombard, New York. These men, together with the seven who signed the letter ("the founder members"), made up the 35 charter members of the Association.

The first meeting of the Association convened on June 2, 1875 in the lecture room of the Young Men's Christian Association Hall at the corner of Fourth Avenue and 23rd Street in New York City (2,3). Eighteen members were present. On the motion of Hammond, Jewell was elected temporary chairman, and he presided at the organizational meeting. The following officers were elected: president, S. Weir Mitchell of Philadelphia; first vice-president, J. S. Jewell of Chicago; second vice-president, E. H. Clarke of Boston; corresponding secretary, J. J. Mason of New York; recording secretary and treasurer, E. C. Seguin of New York; curator, J. W. S. Arnold of New York. Inasmuch as Mitchell, the president-elect, was not present at the meeting, Jewell, the first vice-president, presided at the first session. At the executive session after the morning meeting on the second day, it was announced that a letter had been received from Mitchell regretting his inability to attend and requesting that his name be withdrawn from the list of officers. In his place Jewell was named the first president of the Association, a position which he continued to hold for the next 4 years. It was not until 1910 that Mitchell served as the Association's president.

During the course of the 2-day meeting, 12 scientific papers were presented, covering a wide range of subjects and eliciting lively discussions. The first paper delivered before the Association was by Samuel G. Webber of Boston and was entitled "A Contribution to the Study of Myelitis." Also at this meeting George M. Beard, well known for his interest in neurasthenia and other functional disorders of the nervous system, was elected to membership. Beard was destined to play a short but significant role in the history of the Association.

The second annual meeting was held June 7 and 8, 1876 in the College of Physicians and Surgeons building in New York City, with 16 members present. On the second day Beard gave a paper entitled "The Influence of Mind in the Causation and Cure of Disease and the Potency of Definite Expectation." He stated in this presentation that emotions such as fear, terror, anxiety, and grief might cause disease and that emotions such as reason, hope, joy, resolution, and self-confidence may be used to cure disease. The discussion of this pioneer contribution to psychopathology and psychotherapy was long and involved. Hammond said that if Beard's doctrine was accepted, he "should feel like throwing his diploma away and joining the theologians." Putnam stated that he had never seen any evidence that cure had been effected by mental influence in cases where actual disease existed. Hammond then said that if the idea of Beard were adopted "we should be descending to the level of all sorts of humbuggery." Beard continued to attend the annual meetings of the Association until his untimely death at the age of 46, and made many important contributions to our understanding of the functional disorders of the nervous system.

New members were gradually added to the Association and it continued to have annual meetings at which the attendance was small but fairly consistent. Those taken into the Association during its early years are as follows: George M. Beard of New York in 1875; Eugene Dupuy and Virgil P. Gibney, both of New York, in 1876; Edward C. Spitzka of New York in 1877; Langdon C. Gray of New York in 1878; Royal W. Amidon and William J. Morton, both of New York, in 1879; William Birdsall and Graeme M. Hammond (son of William A. Hammond), both of New York, in 1880; S. V. Clevenger and H. Gradle of Chicago, Charles K. Mills and Wharton Sinkler of Philadelphia, and Burt Wilder of Ithaca, in 1881; Charles L. Dana of New York in 1882; Jeremiah T. Eskridge of Denver in 1883; George W. Jacoby, Ralph L. Parsons, and Leonard Webber, all of New York, and George L. Walton of Boston, in 1884; M. Allen Starr of New York, Philip Zenner of Cincinnati, and Sarah J. McNutt of New York (the first woman to be elected to membership in the Association) in 1885. By the turn of the century its membership included most of the physicians involved in research and treatment of nervous diseases in this country. The second, third, and fourth meetings of the Association were held at the College of Physicians and Surgeons, but subsequent meetings were held in the New York Academy of Medicine. The discussions were interesting, and the early members of the Association were evidently imbued with a deep enthusiasm for their subject. The first 11 meetings of the Association were held in New York City, but the twelfth annual meeting was held in Long Branch, New Jersey. After 1886 the meetings were held in various cities, including Philadelphia, Washington, New York City, Boston, St. Louis, Baltimore, Albany, and Atlantic City. For many years (1932 to 1967) the Association met in Atlantic City with the exception of the following years: in 1940, when Foster Kennedy was president, it met in Rye, New York; in 1946, when Walter Schaller was president, it met in San Francisco; in 1955, when Percival Bailey was president, it met in Chicago; and in 1960, when Derek Denny-Brown was president, it met in Boston. Since 1968 it has met in Washington, Los Angeles, Chicago, Montreal, San Francisco, St. Louis, and Boston.

The first person elected to honorary membership in the Association was

Frederic Bateman of Norwich, England, who was inducted in 1878. In 1881 several honorary memberships were awarded: Jean Martin Charcot of Paris, J. Hughlings Jackson of London, W. H. Erb of Leipzig, Carl Westphal of Berlin, and Theodore Meynert of Vienna. Subsequently elected honorary members during the first 25 years were as follows: William A. Hammond of New York in 1887; Victor Horsley and David Ferrier, both of London, in 1889; S. Weir Mitchell of Philadelphia in 1895; Edward C. Seguin of New York in 1896; William R. Gowers of London and Carl W. H. Nothnagel of Vienna in 1898. William Osler was elected an honorary member in 1905, the year he left Baltimore and went to Oxford. A group of associate members were also elected in 1881: Thomas Dowse of London, Moritz Berhnhardt of Berlin, William R. Gowers of London, David Ferrier of London, Camillo Golgi of Pavia, H. Carlton Bastian of London, J. Russell Reynolds of London, and H. Obersteiner of Vienna. Subsequently elected associate members during the first 25 years were Josial E. Lombard of Norwood, England, in 1881; Auguste Ollivier of Paris in 1882; S. F. Danillo of St. Petersburg and Auguste Forel of Zurich in 1884; H. Mierzejewski of St. Petersburg in 1885; Henri Huchard of Paris in 1890; Arnold Pick of Prague in 1893; and Ludwig Edinger of Frankfurt in 1897. In 1932 the terminology for this category of membership was changed to that of corresponding member, and the category of associate membership was established for nonclinical members.

The American Neurological Association, whose annual meetings are well attended by members and guests, has continued to grow in size and prestige. It has greatly influenced the development of American neurology, and for many decades was the only national neurologic organization. It celebrated its semicentennial anniversary in Philadelphia in 1924 with Charles K. Mills serving his second term as president, and its centennial anniversary in 1975 in New York City with James M. Foley as president. Other neurologic societies have since been formed, but the Association continues as the senior and most respected one.

REFERENCES

1. Denny-Brown, D., Rose, A. S. and Sahs, A. L. (eds.) (1975): *Centennial Anniversary Volume of the American Neurological Association 1875-1975*. Springer, New York.
2. Hunt, J. R. (1924): The foundation and early history of the American Neurological Association. In: *Semi-centennial Anniversary Volume of the American Neurological Association 1875-1924*. pp. 1–15. American Neurological Association, New York.
3. Mills, C. K. (1924): Some recollections of the early meetings and personnel of the American Neurological Association, with a glance at the work of the last fifty years. In: *Semi-Centennial Anniversary Volume of the American Neurological Association 1875–1924*, pp. 16–45. American Neurological Association, New York.

4

American Neurology During the Last Quarter of the Nineteenth Century

During the last quarter of the nineteenth century neurology and psychiatry developed as a dual specialty in the United States as they did in Europe. In most of the medical schools in which these subjects were taught, they were taught together; and most clinicians concerned with these areas dealt with both. However, neurology made more progress as a science during this period than did psychiatry. Physicians dealing with psychiatric patients served more as custodians than as clinicians. In most hopsitals mental patients were separated from other patients, not for diagnosis and treatment, but for the safety of others. They often were segregated, not in hospitals but in asylums which were in part poorhouses and in part jails.

From the time of Benjamin Rush, however, some American physicians did begin to interest themselves in the plight of psychotic patients and tried to improve their condition. This was evident in the establishment of a ward for mental patients in the basement of the Pennsylvania Hospital (where Rush worked) in 1756, and in building a hospital for mental patients at Williamsburg, Virginia, in 1772. In 1818 the McLean Insane Asylum was opened in Massachusetts, followed by the Bloomingdale Asylum in New York in 1821 and the Retreat for the Insane in Hartford, Connecticut, in 1822.

The term psychiatry was not established until the twentieth century. Psychiatrists were initially referred to as alienists. The first name of what was later to be the American Psychiatric Association, organized in 1844, was the Association of Medical Superintendents of American Institutions for the Insane. It was to become the American Medico-Psychological Association in 1894 and finally the American Psychiatric Association in 1921. *The American Journal of Psychiatry* was called the *American Journal of Insanity* from 1844 to 1921.

The demonstration by Duchenne, Erb, and others that nerves and muscles could be stimulated by an electrical current, with a resulting contraction of muscles, led to great interest in the use of electricity in neurologic diagnosis. The earlier users of such electricity also believed it to be of value in treatment as well. James J. Putnam was appointed "electrician" to the Massachusetts General Hospital in 1872, and Samuel G. Webber received a similar appointment at the Boston City Hospital in 1876. Charles K. Mills was appointed lecturer in electrotherapeutics at the University of Pennsylvania in 1877, and William J. Herdman was appointed professor of diseases of the mind and nervous system and electrotherapeutics at the medical department of the University of Michigan in 1892.

American neurology was at first largely concentrated in the eastern states, principally in New York, Philadelphia, and Boston. William A. Hammond and Edward C. Seguin are responsible for introducing neurology into New York City. Seguin was appointed professor of diseases of the nervous system at the College of Physicians and Surgeons in 1870. Hammond was given a similar apointment at the New York University School of Medicine in 1874 and at the Bellevue Hospital Medical College in 1876. These two men were instrumental in the formation of the New York Neurological Society in 1872 and, together with their colleagues in Boston, Philadelphia, Chicago, and other cities, in the formation of the American Neurological Association in 1875. The early development of neurology in New York was centered at the College of Physicians and Surgeons, where Seguin served as professor from 1870 to 1888, when he was succeeded by Moses A. Starr. In 1888 the four sons of William K. Vanderbilt gave funds for the construction of an outpatient building in memory of their father to be annexed to the school. Prior to 1888 neurology had been taught mainly through lectures, but after the establishment of the Vanderbilt Clinic patients were used for teaching. Seguin established and directed the neurology department in the Vanderbilt Clinic and was followed by Starr. Inpatients were cared for in nearby hospitals—New York, Presbyterian, Roosevelt, and St. Luke's Hospitals and later the New York Neurological Institute.

William A. Hammond was professor of diseases of the nervous system at the New York University College of Medicine until 1898. In 1886 Edward G. Janeway was appointed professor of the principles and practice of medicine at the Bellevue Hospital Medical College, where the care of patients with diseases of the nervous system remained under his supervision until 1887. Charles L. Dana then assumed that responsibility until 1898 when the two schools merged. Dana subsequently moved to the newly founded Cornell University Medical College as professor of diseases of the nervous system, and Edward Dix Fisher was named professor of mental and nervous diseases at the New York University College of Medicine and neurologist at Bellevue Hospital, positions he held until 1928. In 1890 twelve beds were assigned to neurology in a new dispensary at Mount Sinai Hospital, and Bernard Sachs was placed in charge of them. For many years Mount Sinai Hospital was affiliated with the College of Physicians and Surgeons, but in 1966 it formed its own medical school, affiliated with the University of the City of New York. In 1884 the Montefiore Home for Chronic Invalids was opened in New

York City. Nineteen of the 44 patients treated there during its first year had chronic neurologic disorders, a figure foreshadowing the later development of a large neurologic service for which the hospital was to become well known. Among the attending physicians during the hospital's early years were Bernard Sachs and Charles L. Dana. Montefiore Hospital was for many years affiliated with the College of Physicians and Surgeons of Columbia University but more recently has been associated with the Albert Einstein School of Medicine.

Many other New York neurologists contributed to the advances of their specialty during the last quarter of the nineteenth century. Some of the more outstanding of them deserve mention:

Landon Carter Gray (1850–1900) was born in New York City (8). He attended Columbia College and then spent 3 years at Heidelberg University, returning to New York and receiving a medical degree from Bellevue Hospital Medical College in 1873. After practicing general medicine for 2 years, he decided to specialize in neurology and within 10 years had achieved an international reputation in this field. In 1883, at the age of 32, he was appointed professor of neurology at the Long Island Hospital College of Medicine, and a few years later he became professor of nervous and mental disease at the New York Polyclinic, where he was a founder of the postgraduate medical school. He was the author of many contributions to neurology and psychiatry, and his *A Treatise on Nervous and Mental Diseases* passed through several editions (14) He was president of the American Neurological Association in 1887.

Edward Charles Spitzka (1852–1914) was a pioneer neurologist and psychiatrist who also made notable contributions to the embryology and comparative anatomy of the nervous system and human neuroanatomy (5). He attended the College of the City of New York and then studied medicine at New York University. After his graduation in 1873 he spent 3 years in Europe, mainly in Berlin, Leipzig, and Vienna, studing embryology, morphology, and psychiatry. He was assistant in embryology at the University of Vienna in 1874 to 1875. He returned to New York City and to practice general medicine but gradually shifted his focus to neurology and psychiatry. He wrote an essay entitled "The Somatic Etiology of Insanity" in which he described the pathologic material gathered from private and public asylums in New York and its environs. This won him a prize offered by the British Medico-Psychological Association in international competition in 1876, and the same year he was the winner of the W. A. Hammond American Neurological Association prize for an essay entitled "The Physiological Effects of Strychnia." He was professor of comparative anatomy in the Columbia University Veterinary College and professor of nervous and mental diseases and of medical jurisprudence at the New York Post-Graduate Medical College from 1882 to 1887. In 1883 he published his book *Insanity: Its Classification, Diagnosis and Treatment*, of which there were two editions (32). Spitzka was president of the American Neurological Association in 1890. He was well known as an expert medical witness, gaining special prominence in his testifying to the insanity of Charles J. Guiteau, the assassin of President James A. Garfield.

Charles Loomis Dana (1852–1935), another of the important pioneers in American neurology, was also known for his literary accomplishments (Fig. 14) (21). He was born in Woodstock, Vermont, and graduated from Dartmouth College in 1872. He served briefly as secretary to the United States senator from Vermont and then as secretary to the director of the Smithsonian Institution. This exposure to natural science led him to enter medical college, and he matriculated in three of them at the same time,

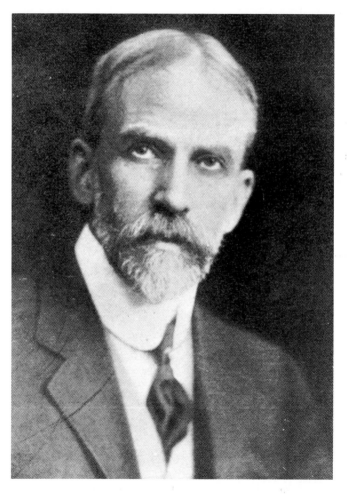

FIG. 14. Charles L. Dana. (From *Arch. Neurol. Psychiatry*, 35:640–646, 1931.)

receiving M.D. degrees from the Columbian Medical College in Washington and the College of Physicians and Surgeons in New York in 1877. He received 2 years of medical training at Bellevue Hospital under Austin Flint and Edward Janeway and throughout his life maintained a connection with that hospital. Shortly after opening an office for the practice of medicine he became interested in diseases of the nervous system. For many years he was responsible for the neurologic service at Bellevue Hospital, which during his lifetime became one of the most important neurologic training centers in the United States.

Dana's first academic appointment was that of professor of physiology at the New York Women's Medical College, a position he held for 3 years. He was professor of diseases of the mind and nervous system at the New York Post-Graduate Hospital from 1884 to 1895. In 1898 he was appointed professor of diseases of the nervous system at the newly founded Cornell University Medical College, a position he held until he retired in 1922, at which time he was named professor emeritus. He was responsible for the inspiration and teaching of two generations of medical students. He was known as a stimulating teacher and a careful clinical investigator, making contributions to our knowledge of epilepsy, narcolepsy, diseases of the basal ganglia, and numerous other neurologic disorders. He first described brain changes due to alcohol and acute transverse myelitis, and with Putnam, was among the first to describe combined sclerosis. He proposed section of the spinal nerve roots for relief of pain and spastic paralysis. His major contribution in the educational field was his *Text Book of Nervous Diseases and Psychiatry for the Use of Students and Practitioners of Medicine* (7), the first edition of which appeared in 1892; 10 editions followed. The book was introduced by a chapter on diagnostic methods and an outline of neurologic diseases. The student was counseled to be aware of the rare diseases but to be thoroughly familiar with the common ones. Dana served as president of the American Neurological Assocation in 1892 and again in 1928.

His literary activities were almost as remarkable as his scientific accomplishments. He, along with neurologists Joseph Collins, Frederick Peterson, and Bernard Sachs, founded the Charaka Club, a literary dining club in New York City. They were joined by other physicians, many of them neurologists. The members presented papers on ancient medicine, on the philosophic, historical, and literary aspects of medicine, as well as on general cultural subjects. These were published in the *Proceedings of the Charaka Club* which appeared at intervals from 1892 to 1947. Among the neurologist members were Mitchell, Pearce Bailey, Smith Ely Jelliffe, and Foster Kennedy; other members who were physicians included John Shaw Billings, Fielding Garrison, George Dock, and Harvey Cushing. William Osler was an honorary member. Dana was also a student of Horace and of medical history, his *Peaks of Medical History* being published in 1926.

Moses Allen Starr (1854–1932) was born in Brooklyn, New York (Fig.

15). During his student years his interests were divided between classical history and natural science. After graduation from Princeton University in 1876 he followed his classical leanings and went to Germany to study Greek and Roman history. After a few visits to Helmholtz's laboratory, however, he began to gravitate to science, and in 1877 he decided to study medicine, his ultimate goal being the study of neurology. Graduating from the College of Physicians and Surgeons in 1880, he served a 2-year residency at Bellevue Hospital, then returning to Europe, where he studied under Erb and Schultze at Heidelberg, Nothnagel and Meynert in Vienna, and Charcot in Paris. Returning to the United States he began his own investigations, and, lacking laboratory facilities, he constructed a laboratory in his home. He studied the sensory pathways and cerebral localization, and in 1888 participated with Ferrier and Horsley in a symposium on the latter subject. He published numerous articles and several books, among which were: *Lectures Upon Diseases of the Mind* (1891), *Lectures Upon Diseases of the Nervous System* (1891), *Familiar Forms of Nervous Disease,* (33) and *Atlas of Nerve Cells* (34). His major text, *Organic and Functional Nervous Dis-*

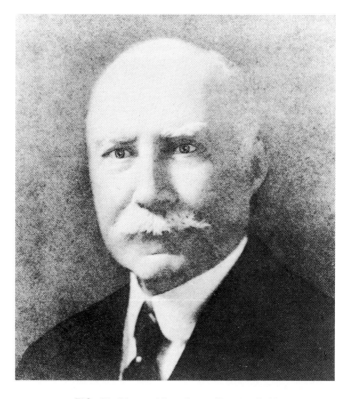

FIG. 15. Moses Allen Starr. (From ref. 1.)

eases (35), was first published in 1903 and went through several editions over the next 10 years.

Starr was professor of nervous diseases at the New York Polyclinic Medical School from 1884 to 1888 and then succeeded Seguin as professor of nervous diseases at the College of Physicians and Surgeons, where he served from 1888 to 1918. He is best remembered as a teacher. Following in the footsteps of Seguin, he, with Dana and Sachs, represented the teaching vanguard of academic neurology in New York. He was president of the American Neurological Association in 1897.

Bernard Sachs (1858–1944) (Fig. 16) was for several decades an outstanding figure in neurology, nationally and internationally (5). He was born in Baltimore and grew up in New York City. He attended Harvard College, from which he graduated in 1878. While there he came under the influence of William James, and as a result developed a keen interest in philosophy and psychology. Through this interest he made an early decision to devote himself to diseases of the mind. Following graduation Sachs enrolled in the new medical center in Strasbourg, from which he graduated in 1882. During the next 2 years he was engaged in postgraduate studies under Meynert in Vienna, Jackson in London, Charcot in Paris, and Westphal in Berlin. He returned to New York to practice in Mount Sinai Hospital but maintained a scholarly interest in neurology. In 1885 he published a translation of Meynert's textbook on psychiatry; that same year he became co-editor of the *Journal of Nervous and Mental Disease* and was its editor from 1886 to 1891. In 1886 he was elected to membership in the American Neurological Association, where he served as president in 1894 and again in 1932.

At the time Sachs joined the staff at the Mount Sinai Hospital, there and elsewhere diseases of the nervous system were treated in the department of medicine. In 1890, however, a new dispensary with nine specialty clinics was organized there. One of these was the neurology clinic, and that year a department of neurology was established with Sachs as head or consultant. In 1900, in recognition of the importance of Sachs' work and of the emergence of neurology as a specialty, the trustees of the Mount Sinai Hospital assigned six beds for men and six for women to the neurology service and designated Sachs chief of the service. For many years this was the only service in New York City that provided facilities for bedside observation of acute neurologic diseases.

In 1887 Sachs published his report "On Arrested Cerebral Development with Special Reference to Its Cortical Pathology." (29) This was the clinicopathologic report of the case of a blind infant with cerebral changes, which he called amaurotic familial idiocy. The ocular manifestations of this condition had been described by a British ophthalmologist, Warren Tay, in 1880, and now it bears the eponym of Tay-Sachs disease. As this report and his other publications indicate, Sachs had an early and persisting interest in pediatric neurology. He contributed studies on intracerebral hemorrhage in

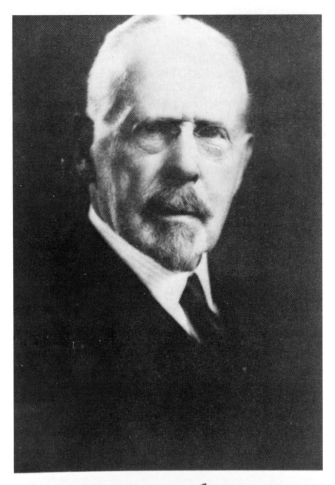

FIG. 16. Bernard Sachs. (From ref. 12.)

the young, cerebral palsy, the muscular dystrophies, and poliomyelitis, as well as on adult neurologic disorders. In 1895 he published his book *Nervous Diseases of Children* (30), and in 1926 with Louis Hausman *Nervous and Mental Disorders from Birth Through Adolesence* (31). He was professor of nervous and mental disease at the New York Polyclinic until 1905. He was appointed professor of clinical neurology at the Columbia University College of Physicians and Surgeons in 1933, director of the division of child neurology at the New York Neurological Institute in 1934, and director of the Child Neurology Research Friedsam Foundation in 1936. He was president of the American Neurological Association in 1894 and 1932.

Following his retirement as chief of the neurology service at the Mount Sinai Hospital in 1924, Sachs devoted himself to the development of international neurology. To this end he met with British and American neurologists in 1927, and in 1928 discussed international neurology with Otto Marburg. Later that year he headed an American committee to plan an international meeting in Switzerland. He was elected president of the First International Neurological Congress which was held in Berne in 1931, and his personal acquaintance with neurologists all over the world, as well as his universal popularity, delicate diplomacy, and personal generosity, contributed to making the Congress a success. He served as honorary president of the next two international congresses. He died at the age of 86 in 1944.

George Miller Beard (1839–1883) was actually more closely allied to psychiatry than to neurology (8). Although a controversial figure, he made significant contributions to the understanding of the so-called functional disturbances of the nervous system and to psychotherapy. He was born in Montville, Connecticut, and attended Yale College, from which he graduated in 1862. In 1966 he graduated from the College of Physicians and Surgeons, at which time he became associated with Alphonso D. Rockwell in the study of nervous diseases and especially in the development of electricity in its relations to medicine and surgery. At the time they began their investigations into electrotherapy, electricity had not been used to any extent by physicians in the United States and only by a few neurologists in Europe. Beard and Rockwell wrote a series of articles on the medical and surgical uses of electricity and finally published their book *A Practical Treatise on the Medical and Surgical Uses of Electricity, Including Localized and Generalized Electrization* in 1871 (4). This was widely read in the United States and abroad, and was translated into several languages. In 1874 Beard established the *Archives of Electrology and Neurology,* which was published semiannually for 2 years.

Beard produced papers on many neurologic subjects but was especially interested in the psychologic and philosophic aspects of nervous diseases. The paper he read before the American Neurological Association in 1876 and the controversy it stimulated are discussed elsewhere. He introduced the concept of neurasthenia, or nervous exhaustion, and in 1880 he published a book on the subject (3). In it he brought to professional attention a large number of symptoms of nervous and functional disease which he contended were of immense importance scientifically and practically. When Thomas Edison thought that he had discovered a new force, the "etheric force," Beard spent much time experimenting on this with Edison and independently, reaching the conclusion that the phenomenon represented an unnoticed phase of induced electricity. Beard's concepts of electrotherapeutics have long since been disproved, as have his philosophic theories of psychodynamics, but he was probably the earliest American psychotherapist. He died in 1883 at the age of 43.

Following the Civil War neurology developed rapidly in Philadelphia, which during the early days was probably the center of neurology in America. It was one of the main centers for the care of the sick and wounded soldiers during the Civil War, and it was in Turner's Lane Hospital, established by Surgeon-General Hammond for the care of patients with nerve injuries and other diseases of the nervous system, that Mitchell, Morehouse, and Keen did their epochal study published as *Gunshot Wounds and Other Injuries of Nerves*. After the war Mitchell continued with his private practice but soon concentrated solely on nervous disorders. He established a teaching clinic for nervous disorders at the Orthopaedic Hospital and Infirmary for Nervous Diseases where he was assisted by Wharton Sinkler. Mitchell interested Osler in joining the staff at the Orthopaedic Hospital, where he shared afternoon clinics with Mitchell and Sinkler for many years. It was from these clinics that he obtained the material for his lectures on chorea and cerebral palsy.

Although a department of neurology was established at the University of Pennsylvania in 1871 with Horatio C. Wood as lecturer on nervous disorders, it was not until Mills was appointed professor of neurology in 1903 that neurology really flourished there. In 1877 a neurology department of 20 beds for men and women was established at the Philadelphia General Hospital, with Mills in charge. In 1878 there were 35 patients in the unit, and by 1910 the number had reached 400. Here Spiller, Dercum, Weisenberg, and a host of others received their training and in turn worked and taught. The Philadelphia General Hospital, with its wealth of acute and chronic neurologic material, was for many years a major American hospital for training in neurology. With the establishment of the Pepper Laboratories in 1895, there were facilities for training in basic neurology as well.

Neurology in Philadelphia, however, soon expanded beyond the University of Pennsylvania, the Orthopaedic Hospital, and the Philadelphia General Hospital. In 1883 a neurology department was established at the Hahnemann Medical College and in 1892 at the Jefferson Medical College. The Philadelphia Neurological Society was established in 1884.

Others who contributed to early neurology in Philadelphia are as follows:

Wharton Sinkler (1845–1910) was born in Philadelphia, but his parents' home was in South Carolina (8). After serving in the Civil War in the South Carolina Cavalry, he enrolled in the University of Pennsylvania Medical School. Following graduation in 1868, he served as house officer at the Episcopal Hospital of Philadelphia, where he later became a member of the visiting staff and a trustee. He was actively connected with the Orthopaedic Hospital and Infirmary for Nervous Diseases for many years, beginning as assistant to Mitchell in 1870. He was a frequent contributor to medical journals from the time of his graduation. His publications on infantile and juvenile paralysis and on infectious and functional nervous diseases were highly regarded. He was especially interested in epilepsy and was instrumental in founding the Pennsylvania Epileptic Hospital and Colony Farm at Oakburn. He was president of the American Neurological Association in 1891.

Francis Xavier Dercum (1858–1920), born in Philadelphia, (8) early became interested in biology. He was graduated from the University of Pennsylvania Medical School in 1877 and the following year received a Ph.D. degree from the same university. He entered private practice but also served as demonstrator in histology and physiology at the University of Pennsylvania. His papers on the sensory organs, the lateral line organs of fish, and the semicircular canals were published as early as 1878 and 1879. His histologic preparations of fungi, protozoa, and bacteria led to contact with bacteriology and pathology, and in 1884 he was appointed consultant pathologist to the State Hospital for the Insane at Norristown. The same year he was also appointed chief of the nervous disease clinic at the University of Pennsylvania and instructor in neurology there. He was appointed professor of nervous and mental diseases at the Jefferson Medical College in 1892 and, from then on, worked there and at the Philadelphia General Hospital. He made many contributions to the neurologic literature and was editor of the *Textbook of Nervous Diseases by American Authors* (1895), which contained chapters by Mitchell, Osler, Dana, Starr, Peterson, and others (9). He described adiposis dolorosa in 1900 (10). As he grew older he became more interested in psychiatry (11) and endocrinology, and published *The Biology of the Internal Secretions* in 1924 (12). He was president of the American Neurological Association in 1896.

In Boston, as was the case elsewhere, it was the skilled and well-rounded physician who first dealt with diseases of the nervous system. James Jackson (1777–1867), professor of the theory and practice of medicine at Harvard Medical School and maternal grandfather of James Jackson Putnam, made an early, concise description of tic douloureux and peripheral neuropathy. He also, in his *Letters to a Young Physician* refers to headache, neuralgia, apoplexy, palsy, and chorea.

Brown-Séquard was achieving widespread recognition as an experimental physiologist and neurologist during the middle decades of the nineteenth century, and on two trips to the United States had given lectures on neurologic subjects that were enthusiastically received in many cities, including Boston. The success of these lectures and the increasing fame of Brown-Séquard were probably what led Harvard Medical School to establish a professorship of physiology and pathology of the nervous system in 1864, which was offered to and accepted by Brown-Séquard. This attempt to establish an academic position in the neurologic sciences did not succeed, however. Brown-Séquard was expected to derive his financial support from the fees for his lectures, and no facilities were available for the continuing of his research. His restless nature and his frequent trips to Europe made it impossible for him to maintain a continuing program. Following the death of his wife in 1867, Brown-Séquard returned to Paris.

Neurology made its first real appearance on the medical scene in Boston in 1872 when Putnam was appointed "electrician" to the Massachusetts General Hospital (8). The next year his title was changed to that of physician to outpatients with diseases of the nervous system. Neurology began at the Boston City Hospital when **Webber** was appointed "electrician" there in 1876, and the next year he was placed in charge of a newly created outpatient department for diseases of the nervous system. It began at Tufts Medical School when Webber was appointed professor of neurology at its opening in 1893. By the end of the century, neurology was flourishing in Boston. Among those, in addition to Putnam, who played important roles in the development of neurology in the Boston area during the last quarter of the nineteenth century are the following:

Samuel G. Webber (1838–1926) was a charter member of the American Neurological Association and delivered the first paper, entitled "A Contribution to the Study of Myelitis," at the first meeting of the Association in 1875 (8). He was a pathologist on the staff of the Boston City Hospital, which had opened its doors in 1864. He showed an early interest in neurologic disease by winning the Boylston Prize at Harvard Medical School with an essay on cerebrospinal meningitis. In 1876 he was appointed "electrician" to the Boston City Hospital and in 1877 was placed in charge of a newly created outpatient department for patients with diseases of the nervous system. Also in 1877 Webber and Robert T. Tedes were appointed visiting physicians for inpatients with diseases of the nervous system, who shared a ward with patients with renal disease. In 1884 he was appointed professor of clinical medicine in the Harvard Medical School, but at the same time beds for neurology were abolished. In 1893, on the opening of Tufts Medical College, he was appointed its first professor of neurology. He published a small book on *Diseases of the Peripheral Cerebro-Spinal Nerves* in 1881.

Robert Thaxter Edes (1838–1923), born in Eastport, Maine, was graduated from Harvard College in 1858 and from Harvard Medical School in 1861. During the Civil War he was an assistant surgeon in the United States Navy. After the war he studied in Europe and on his return practiced general medicine in Boston. He was professor of materia medica (1875–1884) and of clinical medicine (1885–1886) at Harvard Medical School. He was also visiting physician for diseases of the nervous system at the Boston City Hospital. In 1886, in the midst of a promising career, he moved to Washington, D.C. because of his wife's illness. While there he lectured at Columbian University and Georgetown University. After his return to the Boston area he served as resident physician at some private asylums and sanitariums, and then attempted to establish a small private sanitarium of his own. However, after a period of waning success he retired. Edes was president of the American Neurological Association in 1883.

Philip Coombs Knapp (1858–1920), born in Lynn, Massachusetts, graduated from Harvard College in 1878. He then entered Harvard Medical School, from which he graduated in 1883. He served as a house officer in the Boston City Hospital and in the Boston Lunatic Asylum, as it was then called. Between 1887 and 1911 he, with Herman F. Vickery, translated and edited the second and third editions of G. H. von Strumpell's *A Textbook of Medicine for Students and Practitioners,* adding an original chapter on mental diseases to the third edition. His first work as an author was a volume on *The Pathology, Diagnosis and Treatment of Intracranial Masses,* published in 1891 (19). His list of publications covers nearly every aspect of neurology and psychiatry. He was widely known for his knowledge of nervous and mental disease and was often called on as a medicolegal expert. From 1886 until the time of his death he held the position of physician for diseases of the nervous system at the Boston City Hospital and became noted for his skill in diagnosis. He was much interested in the development of his department and had the satisfaction of seeing it grow from a small outpatient clinic to a separate department with special beds for patients with nervous diseases. He believed that mental patients should also be treated on the wards of general hospitals and was instrumental in having this practice adopted at the Boston City Hospital.

The beginnings of neurology were not as auspicious elsewhere along the eastern seaboard. Francis T. Miles, the second president of the American Neurological Association (in 1880) was appointed clinical professor of diseases of the nervous system and professor of general, descriptive, and surgical anatomy at the University of Maryland in Baltimore in 1869. In 1880 he abandoned anatomy and became professor of physiology, but remained clinical professor of diseases of the nervous system until his retirement in 1903. He was a popular teacher and physician. He conducted a teaching clinic on nervous diseases one day a week.

At the Medical College of Virginia in Richmond, Brown-Séquard held the post of professor of the institutes of medicine (now the chair of physiology) for a short time in 1854. At the University College of Medicine, also in Richmond, J. Allison Hodges was professor of nervous diseases from 1896 until 1910, when the college merged with the Medical College of Virginia. At the Medical College of South Carolina in Charleston, Samuel Henry Dickson, professor of the institutes and practice of physic, published his textbook *Elements of Medicine* in 1859. It contained a 49-page section on "Diseases of the Sensorial System." Eugene D. Bondurant was appointed professor of neurology and psychiatry in the department of medicine of the University of Alabama in Mobile in 1897. A graduate of the University of

Virginia who had studied in Heidelberg, Vienna, and London, he wrote on neurologic subjects including poliomyelitis, neuritis (3), beriberi, chorea, and neurosyphilis.

Neurology developed early in upstate New York. Henry Hun (1854–1924) was appointed professor of neurology at the Albany Medical College in 1885. Born in Albany, the son of one of the founders of the Albany Medical College, Hun was graduated from Harvard Medical School in 1879 and then spent 2 years in Vienna, Heidelberg, Berlin, Paris, and London. He received his academic appointment on his return to Albany and continued in this position until 1914. Hun's influence on medical students was profound and lasting. He was the author of numerous articles, and his book *An Atlas of the Differential Diagnosis of Diseases of the Nervous System* was published in 1913 (18). His description of the lateral medullary syndrome is classic. He was president of the American Neurological Association in 1914.

James Wright Putnam (1860–1938) served as professor of neurology at the University of Buffalo from 1891 to 1922. Putnam made some notable contributions to the neurologic literature, particularly a report of a case of athetosis with autopsy. He was president of the American Neurological Association in 1903.

In the Middle West neurology gained the most prominence in Chicago and St. Louis. Roberts Bartholow, the third president of the American Neurological Association, was the first person to stimulate the waking human brain. He did this in Cincinnati in 1874 but shortly thereafter moved to Philadelphia. During a long career Frank W. Langdon was first a professor of anatomy (1884–1895) and then of nervous and mental diseases at the University of Cincinnati (1895–1918). He had studied with Gowers in London. Henry Upson was the professor of nervous and mental diseases at Western Reserve University Medical School in Cleveland from 1895 to 1912. In Minnesota Charles Eugene Riggs was appointed professor of mental and nervous disease at the St. Paul Medical College in 1882 and in 1888 became professor at the newly organized University of Minnesota. Riggs was considered the first neurologist in the Northern Midwest. William Alexander Jones held the title of adjunct professor of nervous and mental diseases at the University of Minnesota and in 1893 was appointed full professor. He was the founder of the Minnesota Neurological Society in 1909. Although residents of New Orleans, Louisiana, and Knoxville, Tennessee, are listed as charter members of the American Neurological Association, there was no activity of record in either of these cities during the nineteenth century.

Neurology evolved in Chicago during the period from 1850 to 1875 (20). James S. Jewell, the first president of the American Neurological Association and remaining in that position for its first 5 years, was a resident of Chicago. With Henry Martyn Bannister he founded the *Chicago Journal of Nervous and Mental Disease*, which 2 years later became the *Journal of Nervous and Mental Disease*. Jewell was a scholarly and influential pioneer of neurology in Chicago. He was a facile writer and thought-provoking speaker.

Bannister (1844–1920) was born in Cazenovia, New York, and received degrees of Ph.B. and A.M. from Northwestern University. He worked for 5 years as a geologist before entering the study of medicine. He was graduated from the National Medical College in Washington, D.C. in 1871. He was a charter member of the American Neurological Association and the Chicago Neurological Society. He gave up his editorial position in 1860 when he moved to Kankakee, Illinois, to become assistant superintendent of the state hospital there. He suffered severely from arthritis deformans and during the last 14 years of his life was an invalid restricted to his home in Evanston, Illinois.

Walter Hay (1830–1875) was born in Georgetown, D.C., and was graduated from the Columbian Medical College there in 1853. Four years later he moved to Chicago and set up a practice in neuropsychiatry that was to continue for 36 years. He joined the faculty of Rush Medical College and was active in organizing St. James Episcopal and St. Luke's Hospitals. He helped to establish the Chicago Department of Health in 1867, and in 1871 organized the department of nervous and mental diseases at Rush Medical College; 2 years later he formed a similar department in St. Joseph's Hospital. Along with Jewell and Bannister he was a charter member of the American Neurological Association. In 1882 he left Rush Medical College to join the faculty at the Northwestern University School of Medicine as professor of materia medica and therapeutics. Upon the retirement of Jewell in 1884, Hay became professor of nervous and mental disease and of medical jurisprudence.

Henry Munson Lyman (1835–1902), one of the most scholarly members of the medical profession in Chicago, was born in Hawaii. He was graduated from Williams College and in 1861 from the College of Physicians and Surgeons; two years later he started a practice in Chicago. Lyman held numerous hospital appointments. He served as professor of physiology and of diseases of the nervous system at Rush Medical College from 1877 to 1890 and was the first person to give instruction in clinical (versus didactic) neurology at the medical school. From 1890 to 1900 he was professor of the principles and practice of medicine at Rush. He also held this position at the Woman's Medical College from 1880 to 1888. He became a member of the American Neurological Association in 1887 and served as its president in 1893. He is especially known for his contributions to the neurologic and general medical literature. *A Treatise on the Theory and Practice of Medicine* was published in 1892, and he also wrote a chapter on disorders of sleep in Pepper's *System of Medicine*, a monograph on anesthesia, and many articles on neurologic subjects.

Daniel Roberts Brower (1839–1909) was graduated from the medical department of Georgetown University in 1864. After serving in the United

States Army and as superintendent of the Eastern Lunatic Asylum of Virginia at Williamsburg, he moved to Chicago to practice neurology and psychiatry. He was professor of mental diseases, materia medica, and therapeutics at Rush Medical College from 1891 to 1899 as well as neurologist at St. Joseph's and Cook County Hospitals and attending physician at Woman's and Presbyterian Hospitals.

Neurology developed rapidly in Chicago during the last quarter of the nineteenth century, a growth that culminated in the founding of the Chicago Neurological Society on January 5, 1898. This act of organization united the city's individual neurologists into a cohesive and continuing group. Many neurologists (most of whom also practiced psychiatry and general medicine) were active during this period, among whom were Richard Smith Dewey, Daniel Roberts Brown, Shobal Vail Clevenger, Harold N. Moyer, Oscar A. King, and James G. Kiernan. Moreover, others who were to become prominent in the field of neurology during the first quarter of the next century were beginning to make contributions to neurology. These include Julius Grinker, George W. Hall, Hugh T. Patrick, Archibald Church, and Sanger Brown.

St. Louis has long been an important center for the neurologic sciences. In 1880 two St. Louis neurologists and psychiatrists, Jerome K. Bauduy and Charles H. Hughes, founded the journal *Alienist and Neurologist,* which continued publication for 40 years.

James K. Bauduy (1842–1914) was born in Cuba (8). He received his classical education at Georgetown College and the University of Louvain, and he was graduated from the Jefferson Medical College in 1865. After serving in the Civil War he settled in St. Louis and established a practice in neurology and psychiatry. He served for a time as consulting physician to the St. Louis Hospital for the Insane and for 25 years was chief physician to St. Vincent's Hospital for the Insane. He was professor of nervous and mental diseases and of medical jurisprudence at the Missouri Medical College for 30 years. This college later became the Washington University School of Medicine. At the time of his death he was professor emeritus of psychologic medicine and diseases of the nervous system at Washington University. His book *Lectures on Diseases of the Nervous System,* published in 1876 (2), is a comprehensive review of the neurology and psychiatry of that time. He wrote many papers on neurologic subjects and was a fluent teacher. He was one of the founding members of the American Neurological Association.

Charles H. Hughes (1839–1916) was graduated from Grinnell College and then from the St. Louis Medical College in 1859. He served in the Civil War through 1865. In 1866 he was appointed superintendent of the Missouri State Lunatic Asylum at Fulton, where he remained for 5 years. He was one of the founders of the Marion Sims Medical College in St. Louis and was its first president and first professor of nervous and mental diseases. This college later was incorporated into the St. Louis University School of Medicine. Charles G. Chaddock, whose important work was to be done during the next century, succeeded Hughes as professor of nervous and mental diseases in the St. Louis University School of Medicine in 1892.

Frank Fry was the first professor of diseases of the nervous system at the Washington University School of Medicine. Like many others, he also taught anatomy. When he retired he was suceeded by Sidney Schwab, whose major contributions to neurology were to be made during the next century.

Neurology at the University of Michigan in Ann Arbor had its beginnings in 1888, at which time William J. Herdman was appointed professor of practical anatomy and diseases of the nervous system in the Department of Medicine and Surgery (the title of the University of Michigan Medical School from its founding in 1850 until its present title was adopted in 1915). Herdman (1848–1896) was a University of Michigan graduate, having received a Ph.B. degree in 1872 and an M.D. degree 1875. Following graduation he had served on the faculty of his alma mater successively as a demonstrator of anatomy, lecturer and later assistant professor of pathologic anatomy, and professor of practical and pathological anatomy between the years 1875 and 1888. His title of professor of practical anatomy and diseases of the nervous system was changed to that of professor of diseases of the mind and nervous system in 1890, thus separating the clinical discipline from anatomy. In 1892 his title was again changed, to that of professor of diseases of the mind and nervous system and electrotherapeutics, which appointment he held until his premature death in 1906. For a time he also held the title of professor of railway injuries in the Law Department of the University of Michigan.

Nearby, the Detroit College of Medicine was established in 1885 by the union of the Detroit Medical College (founded in 1868) and the Medical College of Michigan (founded in 1879). From its beginning, the Detroit College of Medicine had a department of diseases of the nervous system, with David Inglis as professor of nervous and mental disease and F. P. Anderson as professor of diseases of the nervous system. Inglis, who had graduated from the Detroit Medical College in 1871 and Bellevue Hospital Medical College in 1872, had been on the faculty of the Detroit Medical College since 1879, serving first as instructor in chemistry and physiology, then as instructor in the practice of medicine, and later as professor of the principles and practice of medicine. Anderson's name does not appear in the bulletins of either the Detroit Medical College or the Michigan College of Medicine. In 1888 his title at the Detroit College of Medicine was changed to that of professor of physiology. Inglis continued on the faculty of the Detroit College of Medicine and its successor, the Detroit College of Medicine and Surgery, until his retirement in 1919. In 1893 his title was changed to professor of clinical neurology and in 1901 to professor of mental and nervous diseases. His interests were more closely allied to psychiatry than to neurology.

There was little spread of neurology west of the Mississippi River prior to the turn of the century. Even though Los Angeles and San Francisco, as well as Denver, Seattle, and Portland, and, closer to the Mississippi River, Rochester, Minnesota, were all to become prominent neurologic centers during the twentieth century, neither neurology nor psychiatry received much prominence in them during the earlier years.

No history of American neurology during the latter part of the nineteenth century would be complete without including that great internist **William Osler** (1849–1919). Born in Bond Head, Ontario, Canada, he graduated from the McGill University Faculty of Medicine and was professor of medicine at his alma mater from 1874 to 1884. He was then professor of medicine at the University of Pennsylvania School of Medicine from 1884 to 1889 and at the Johns Hopkins University School of Medicine from 1889 to 1905, when he was appointed Regius Professor of Medicine at Oxford University. He was later to be knighted and become Sir William Osler.

Osler was very much interested in clinical neurology and diseases of the nervous system. During his many European trips he attended the lectures of Dejerine, Charcot, Marie, and other French and German neurologists. His close friends included Mitchell and Cushing in America as well as most of the leading English neurologic scientists: Ferrier, Horsley, Sherrington, and Gowers. In 1888 he gave a series of three lectures on cerebral localization in Toronto which were enthusiastically received. While in Philadelphia he worked with Mitchell at the Orthopaedic Hospital and Infirmary for Nervous Diseases. His monographs *The Cerebral Palsies of Children* (1889) (25) and *On Chorea and Choreiform Affections* (1894) (26) were written from his experiences there. Among his neurologic contributions are papers on cerebral hemorrhage, concussion, brain tumors, aneurysms, cerebral embolism, poliomyelitis, and meningitis. His *The Principles and Practice of Medicine* (27), which was first published in 1892 and went through many revisions, was the best known textbook on the subject of its time. His extensive section on "Diseases of the Nervous System" was outstanding. Although basically an internist, Osler should be placed among the foremost American neurologists of the period. He also made many contributions to the history of medicine and on his death bequeathed his remarkable collection of important historical medical books to McGill University.

The first recorded lumbar (or spinal) puncture done on a living person was by an American investigator (14). In 1885 J. Leonard Corning, a New York physician, showed that a needle can be inserted between the spinous processes of the lumbar vertebrae and into the subarachnoid space without prior removal of the arches of the vertebrae (6). His purpose was to inject cocaine hydrochlorate into the subarachnoid space to produce spinal anesthesia, and he performed it first on a dog and then on a man. Lumbar punctures for the removal of cerebrospinal fluid (CSF) were subsequently performed by Morton (24) and Wynter (36) in England and by Quincke (28) in Keil, Germany, in 1891. The first two investigators drained the CSF in patients with tuberculous meningitis, incising the skin and using a trocar and cannula. Quincke, like Corning, introduced the needle without incising the skin (13).

NEUROLOGY EDUCATION AND PRACTICE

During the last quarter of the nineteenth century, medicine and medical schools, and with them neurology, continued to spread throughout the country. Many of the medical schools, rapidly proliferating, were private or proprietary schools, and for the most part were small and short-lived. Departments of nervous and mental disease (or of diseases of the mind and nervous system) were established at most of the larger schools and especially at those associated with universities. Often the term "electrotherapeutics" was included in the department's title. Teaching consisted of a series of lectures, as bedside teaching was not in use until well into the twentieth century. Moreover, there were no programs for postgraduate instruction in diseases of the nervous system.

During this period neurology and psychiatry were practiced together, and many practitioners who called themselves neurologists practiced more psychiatry than neurology. There was little specific therapy for disorders of the nervous system: Bromides were used for epilepsy, but most of the other pharmaceutical agents used were given empirically.

Research into the basic neurosciences had its beginnings in America during this period. **Burt Green Wilder** (1841–1925), who was professor of physiology, vertebrate zoology, and neurology at Cornell University in Ithaca, New York for many years, took a special interest in neuroanatomy (23). He expressed the belief that there was need for comparative studies of the brains of talented persons, criminals, the mentally ill, and suicides, but did no neuropathology himself. He had many interests, and his neuroanatomic publications are few. He was president of the American Neurological Association in 1885.

Among the others who made contributions to neuroanatomy and comparative neurology during this period are Donaldson and the Herrick brothers. **Henry Herbert Donaldson** (1857–1938) was assistant professor of neurology (neuroanatomy) at the University of Chicago from 1892 to 1906, and director of research at the Wistar Institute from 1906 until his retirement (22). He conducted important investigations in comparative neuroanatomy but is best known for the part he played in developing a specific breed of albino rats as a valuable laboratory standard. He was president of the American Neurological Association in 1937.

Clarence Luther Herrick (1858–1904) embarked on a program of research in comparative neurology and psychology after having served for 10 years on a geological and natural history survey of Minnesota. In 1891 he established and became the first editor of the *Journal of Comparative Neurology*, which was published first in Cincinnati and then, beginning in 1892, at Denison University in Granville, Ohio. In 1893 he developed acute pulmonary tuberculosis and had to give up his editorial duties. He moved to New Mexico. His younger brother, **Charles Judson Herrick** (1868–1960)

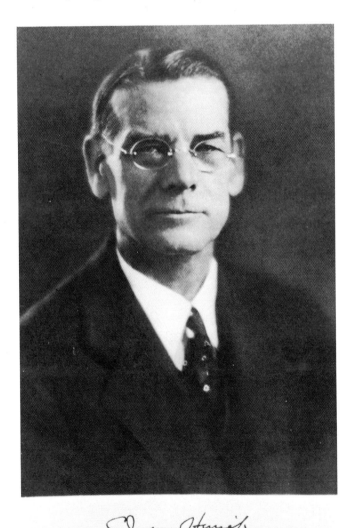

FIG. 17. C. Judson Herrick. (Courtesy of Elizabeth C. Crosby.)

(Fig. 17), assumed the responsibilities for the journal, and at Clarence Herrick's death in 1904 assumed the position of editor, which he continued to hold until the journal was acquired by the Wistar Institute in 1908 (1). He continued to serve on the editorial board, however, until his retirement, when he was named editor emeritus. In 1908 C. Judson Herrick succeeded Donaldson as professor of neurology (neuroanatomy) at the University of Chicago where he remained until his retirement. He made many important contributions to comparative neuroanatomy, and many eminent neuroanatomists received their training under him (15). Over a period of 40 years he collaborated with George E. Coghill, then at the Wistar Institute, in his investigations. Coghill, too, had been stimulated to study comparative neurology by Clarence Herrick. C. Judson Herrick's textbook, *Introduction to Neurology* (16) was a classic and went through many editions. His most important writings are incorporated into *The Evolution of Human Nature*, in which he gave his final reflections on the "big problems of the meaning of life." He published *The Thinking Machine* in 1922 (17).

Clinical research made more progress during this period than basic research and consisted mainly of detailed descriptions of the symptoms, signs, and clinical courses of neurologic diseases by Mills, Putnam, Seguin, Dana, Huntington, and others. Also to be included with clinical research is the study of the stimulation of the living human brain by Bartholow.

REFERENCES

1. Bailey, P. (1975): Moses Allan Starr 1854–1932. In: *Centennial Anniversary Volume of the American Neurological Association 1875–1975*, edited by D. Denny-Brown, A. S. Rose, and A. L. Sahs, pp. 112–113. Springer, New York.
2. Bauduy, J. K. (1876): *Lectures on Diseases of the Nervous System.* Lippincott, Philadelphia.
3. Beard, G. M. (1880): *A Practical Treatise on Nervous Exhaustion (Neurasthenia).* William Wood & Co., New York.
4. Beard, G. M., and Rockwell, A. D. (1871): *A Practical Treatise on the Medical and Surgical Uses of Electricity, Including Localized and Generalized Electrization* William Wood & Co., New York.
5. Bender, M. B. (1975): Bernard Sachs 1858–1944. In: *Centennial Anniversary Volume of the American Neurological Association 1875–1975*, edited by D. Denny Brown, A. S. Rose, and A. L. Sahs, pp. 102–107. Springer, New York.
6. Corning, J. L. (1885): Spinal anesthesia and local medication to the cord. *New York Med. J.*, 42:483–487.
7. Dana, C. L. (1892): *A Textbook of Nervous Diseases and Psychiatry for the Use of Students and Practitioners of Medicine.* William Wood & Co., New York.
8. Denny-Brown, D., Rose, A. S., and Sahs, A. L. (eds.) (1975): *Centennial Anniversary Volume of the American Neurological Association 1875–1975.* Springer, New York.
9. Dercum, F. X. (ed.) (1895): *A Textbook on Nervous Diseases by American Authors.* Lea Brothers & Co., Philadelphia.
10. Dercum, F. X. (1900): Autopsy in a case of adiposis dolorosa with microscopical examination. *J. Nerv. Ment. Dis.*, 27:419–429.
11. Dercum, F. S. (1913): *Clinical Manual of Mental Disease.* Saunders, Philadelphia.
12. Globus, J. H. (1953): Bernard Sachs (1858–1944). In: The Founders of Neurology, edited by W. Haymaker, pp. 376–379. Charles C Thomas, Springfield, Illinois.

13. Gray, H. (1921): A history of lumbar puncture (rachientesis): The operation and the idea. *Arch. Neurol. Psychiatry*, 6:61–69.
14. Gray, L. C.: *A Treatise on Nervous and Mental Diseases for Students and Practitioners of Medicine*. Lea Brothers & Co., Philadelphia.
14a. Haymaker, W., ed. (1953): *The Founders of Neurology*. Charles C Thomas, Springfield, Illinois.
15. Herrick, C. J. (1948): *Brain of the Tiger Salamander*. University of Chicago Press, Chicago.
16. Herrick, C. J. (1918): *Introduction to Neurology*. Saunders, Philadelphia.
17. Herrick, C. J. (1922): *The Thinking Machine*. University of Chicago Press, Chicago.
18. Hun, H. (1915): *An Atlas of the Differential Diagnosis of Diseases of the Nervous System*. The Southworth Company, Troy, New York.
19. Knapp, P. C. (1891): *The Pathology, Diagnosis and Treatment of Intra-Cranial Masses*. Press of Rockwell and Churchill. Boston.
20. Mackay, R. P. (1964): The history of neurology in Chicago. *Illinois Med. J.*, 125:51–58, 142–146, 256–259, 341–344, 539–544, 636–640; 126:60–64.
21. McDowell, F., and Denny-Brown, D. (1975): Charles L. Dana 1852–1935. In: *Centennial Anniversary Volume of the American Neurological Association 1875–1975*, edited by D. Denny-Brown, A. S. Rose, and A. L. Sahs, pp. 96–101. Springer, New York.
22. Mettler, F. A. (1975): Henry Herbert Donaldson, 1857–1938. In: *Centennial Anniversary Volume of the American Neurological Association 1875–1975*, edited by D. Denny-Brown, A. S. Rose, and A. L. Sahs, pp. 205–210. Springer, New York.
23. Mettler, F. A. (1975): Burt Green Wilder 1841–1925. In: *Centennial Anniversary Volume of the American Neurological Association 1875–1975*, edited by D. Denny-Brown, A. S. Rose, and A. L. Sahs, pp. 75–80. Springer, New York.
24. Morton, C. A. (1891): The pathology of tuberculous meningitis, with reference to treatment by tapping the subarachnoid space of the spinal cord. *Br. Med. J.*, 2:840–843.
25. Osler, W. (1889): *The Cerebral Palsies of Children*. Blakiston, Philadelphia.
26. Osler, W. (1894): *On Chorea and Choreiform Affections*. Blakiston, Philadelphia.
27. Osler, W. (1892): *The Principles and Practice of Medicine*. Appleton, New York.
28. Quincke, H. (1891): Die Lumbalponction des Hydrocephalus. *Berl. Klin. Wochenschr.*, 28:529–539.
29. Sachs, B. (1887): On arrested cerebral development with special reference to its cortical pathology. *J. Nerv. Ment. Dis.*, 13:541–553.
30. Sachs, B. (1895): *Nervous Diseases of Children*. William Wood & Co., New York.
31. Sachs, B., and Hausman, L. (1926): *Nervous and Mental Disorders from Birth Through Adolescence*. Hoeber, New York.
32. Spitzka, E. C. (1887): *Insanity: Its Classification, Diagnosis and Treatment*. E. B. Trent, New York.
33. Starr, M. A. (1870): *Familiar Forms of Nervous Diseases*. William Wood & Co., New York.
34. Starr, M. A. (1870): *Atlas of Nerve Cells*. Macmillan, New York.
35. Starr, M. A. (1903): *Organic and Functional Nervous Diseases*. Lea Brothers & Co., Philadelphia.
36. Wynter, W. E. (1891): Four cases of tubercular meningitis in which paracentesis of the theca vertebralis was performed for the relief of fluid pressure. *Lancet*, 1:981–983.

5

American Neurology During the First Quarter of the Twentieth Century

At the onset of the twentieth century there were no institutions in the United States for the care and treatment of patients with diseases of the nervous system; and only a very few hospitals (e.g., Mount Sinai Hospital in New York and Philadelphia General Hospital) had special wards for these patients. Individuals with nervous system disorders were usually placed in general medical wards and were cared for by general practitioners or internists, who, if they deemed it necessary, called a neurologist in consultation. If an operation on the brain or spinal cord was thought to be advisable, a general surgeon was called on to perform it. There were neurology departments in many outpatient clinics, however, and young physicians who wished to become proficient in the field of diseases of the nervous system were forced to gain most of their experience in these clinics and by studying their own private patients. A few were fortunate enough to act as assistants to older neurologists and help them in their consultations on hospital wards.

It became apparent to many thoughtful neurologists that the establishment of special wards for the care of patients with diseases of the nervous system was necessary and would serve two important purposes: It would provide facilities for improved patient care and an environment for the training of young neurologists. It was recognized only later that such wards would also aid in more rapid dissemination of knowledge of the specialty and provide facilities for research on the nervous system and its diseases.

THE FOUNDING AND EARLY HISTORY OF THE NEUROLOGICAL INSTITUTE OF NEW YORK

Early in 1909 two New York neurologists, Joseph Collins and Joseph Fraenkel, became convinced that there was need for a special hospital to be devoted entirely to the study and treatment of patients with diseases of the nervous system, and on March 9, 1909, Collins sent the following letter to a group of prominent businessmen who were friends of his: (46)

My dear _____,

Dr. Joseph Fraenkel and I have for a long time been nurturing plans for the establishment in NewYork of a small hospital for the study and treatment of nervous diseases, particularly the so-called functional varieties including brief and curable mental disorders. We think that the time has come to proceed to the maturation of these plans. We would like very much to get expressions of opinion from a few men of affairs concerning the best way to proceed with the establishment of such a hospital, its location, method of administration, etc. Will you do me the honor to dine with me at the Century Club, 7 West 43rd Street, Thursday evening, March 18th at 7:30?

In addition to Collins and Fraenkel, the following were present at the dinner: Robert P. Perkins, Richard H. Williams, Isaac Townsend, Otto H. Kahn, Paul Warburg, Adrian Iselin Jr., H. K. Knapp, and Dr. Lightner Witmer. After the dinner Collins and Fraenkel explained the object of the meeting and obtained an enthusiastic response. It was felt that the plans should be carried out, and those present agreed to act as founders until a board of trustees had been organized (81,89).

Collins and Fraenkel then had a series of meetings, in one of which they decided to ask another New York neurologist, Pearce Bailey, to join them. The three of them then met on numerous occasions and came to the decision that the hospital should be founded immediately and that it was necessary to ask several wealthy men to help them. Collins offered to write articles of incorporation and look for a building to be rented or bought. He stated that he would drop his other hospital connections in order to devote all of his time to the hew hospital which, at his suggestion, was to be called the Neurological Institute of New York. It was decided that each of the men present at the dinner, except the physicians, be a trustee; also named as trustees were Isaac Seligman, Richard W. Gilder, and George Frelinghuysen.

During further discussions it was suggested that a neurosurgeon be asked to join them, and Charles A. Elsberg, an enthusiastic proponent of the future of neurosurgery in America, was invited to the next meeting. It was further suggested that Bailey, Collins, and Fraenkel be named physicians, and Elsberg surgeon, to the Institute. At the close of one meeting Bailey said, "Before we adjourn, may I say to you that I am deeply impressed at the conclusions that we have reached this evening. I believe that this is pioneer work, and that if we succeed, future generations will call us pioneers and that before long other neurological institutes will be founded in this country and other parts of the world." One wonders if he were not aware of the existence of the National Hospital for the Paralyzed and Epileptic, Queen Square, in London, and the Salpêtrière in Paris.

Articles of incorporation were signed on April 14, 1909, and a vacant six-story building at 149 East 67 Street was leased for 2.5 years. This had formerly been the outpatient department and nurses' home of Mount Sinai Hospital, and could easily be remodeled to serve the purposes of the Institute. There was no formal opening of the building: As soon as structural alterations had been completed and apparatus had been installed, the hospital was declared open. The first outpatients were seen on November 19, 1909, and on December 2 the first patients were admitted to the hospital. Ten days later there were 25 patients in the wards and private rooms.

The first staff of the Institute consisted of Bailey, Collins, and Fraenkel (attending neurologists) and Elsberg (attending neurosurgeon), with Charles L. Dana and Bernard Sachs as consultants in neurology. In 1911, however, some of the members of the medical staff began openly to criticize the management of the hospital and thought that private patients should not be cared for in the Institute. These matters were thoroughly discussed at meetings of the Board of Trustees and the Medical Board, but no agreement was reached. As a consequence Fraenkel severed his connections with the Institute during its second year, taking with him several of the wealthiest and most generous members of the Board of Trustees. Soon thereafter Frederick Peterson was appointed to the staff in Fraenkel's place, and Charles L. Dana was elected to the Board of Trustees. Under Bailey, Collins, Dana, and Peterson, the Institute was reorganized, new members were elected to the Board of Trustees, and a threatened closing of the Institute was forestalled.

Shortly after the reorganization Alfred B. Taylor was appointed associate surgeon, and over the next several years many more physicians and surgeons were appointed to the staff, among whom were Samuel Brock, Louis Casamajor, Thomas K. Davis, Cornelius Dyke, J. Ramsay Hunt, Smith Ely Jelliffe, Foster Kennedy, Henry A. Riley, Byron Stookey, Frederick Tilney, Walter Timme, and Edwin G. Zabriskie. There were also junior staff members and physicians in training. The Institute became an important research and teaching center, and was visited by increasing numbers of American and foreign neurologists.

Soon after the Congress of the United States declared war on Germany, the Surgeon General's office asked the Neurological Institute if it was willing to turn over the hospital for use by the War Department. The Board of Trustees and Medical Board thought that it should continue in its civilian status but offered its services for the treatment of military personnel with injuries and diseases of the nervous system (46).

During the First World War the staff of the Institute was greatly depleted, as 30 members of the medical staff entered military service, including Drs. Bailey and Collins. At the request of the Surgeon General of the United States Army, courses for medical officers were held at the Institute, with Walter Timme in charge. In addition, Elsberg was asked to direct a school for instruction of medical officers in neurosurgery.

After the war it became increasingly evident that the facilities of the Institute were inadequate. The number of outpatients and hospitalized patients was excessive, and the facilities for neurosurgery and postoperative care were meager. Increased space was needed for laboratories, research, and teaching. Purchase of the Polyclinic Hospital, which at that time was used as a veterans' hospital, was considered but soon given up. At about that time a letter was received from Nicholas Murray Butler, president of Columbia University, concerning a possible affiliation between the Institute and the university. In December 1919 the resignations of Bailey, Collins, and Peterson as attending physicians were accepted by the Board of Trustees; they were then appointed consulting physicians, and Edwin G. Zabriskie, Foster Kennedy, and Walter Timme were elected attending physicians. These three neurologists and Elsberg, the neurosurgeon, constituted the Medical Board. In the fall of 1919 the owner of the building informed the Medical Board that their lease would not be renewed after April 1, 1920, as he wished to sell the building. Confronted by this emergency, the four members of the Medical Board proposed a plan for purchasing the building. They would personally contribute $17,500 if the additional amount requred for the purchase of the building could be raised by the Board of Trustees. On February 3, 1920, the building was purchased for $180,000. Important and much needed improvements to the building were then made at an additional cost of $40,000. A realignment of the beds in the hospital was made and a fourth medical service added. Frederick Tilney, professor of neurology at the College of Physicians and Surgeons of Columbia University, was appointed attending physician and placed in charge of this service.

For a number of years it had been evident to those who had the future of the Neuological Institute at heart that it could not continue in its inadequate quarters, and that if the demands made on it were to be satisfied a modern building and equipment were necessary. After prolonged discussion and serious consideration of many alternatives, the Board of Trustees and the Medical Board concluded that the Institute should be affiliated with the College of Physicians and Surgeons of Columbia University and the Columbia-Presbyterian Medical Center. This affiliation was completed in 1925, and the Institute moved into its new building on the corner of 168th Street and Fort Washington Avenue in 1929.

Founders of the Neurological Institute

Pearce Bailey (1865–1922) (Fig. 18), born in New York City (5), was graduated from Princeton University and the College of Physicians and Surgeons of Columbia University. Following an internship at St. Luke's Hospital in New York City, he spent 2 years in Europe, mainly in Paris, Berlin, and Munich, intensively studying the normal and diseased nervous system. On his return from Europe he joined Starr at the Vanderbilt Clinic and entered private practice. He served as adjunct professor of neurology at the College of Physicians and Surgeons from 1906 to 1910. His early writings dealt mainly with neuropathologic and neurologic problems. His book *Accident and Injury: Their Relation to Diseases of the Nervous System*, which

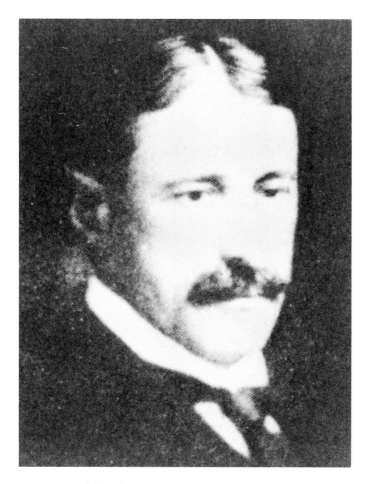

FIG. 18. Pearce Bailey. (From ref. 43.)

was first published in 1898, went through several editions. He was a gifted organizer and played an important part in establishing two landmarks in American neurology. In 1909, with Joseph Collins, he founded the Neurological Institute of New York, the first hospital for neurologic diseases in America. In 1917 he, with Stewart Paton and Thomas Salmon, comprised an informal committee to establish plans for screening military inductees and to supervise the management of neurologic and psychiatric casualties at home and abroad. Their suggestions were accepted by Surgeon General Gorgas, who asked Bailey to organize a division of psychiatry and neurology in the medical department of the United States Army. When Bailey retired from the army he was awarded the Distinguished Service Medal by the United States Congress. After World War I he gave much of his time to the

New York State Commission for Mental Deficiency, of which he was chairman. He established the Classification Clinic at the Neurological Institute, which was later known as the Child Guidance Clinic. He also had a keen literary interest, and wrote many stories, skits, and plays. His psychological study "Voltaire's Relation to Medicine" was well received. Bailey was a charter member of the Charaka Club and was president of the American Neurological Association in 1913.

Bailey was an attractive man, tall and stately, careful of speech, and able to express himself forcefully. During the development of the Neurological Institute he gave unstintingly of his time and energy. His rounds with his staff were always well attended; he was an exponent not only of the art of neurology but the art of teaching as well. He was a man of many interests with a wide knowledge of general literature as well as of neurology. He died of pneumonia at the age of 57.

Joseph Collins (1866–1950) (Fig. 19) achieved renown as a neurologist and an author of popular books (72). He was born in Brookfield, Connecticut, and during his early life had problems with poverty and ill health. He attended the University of Michigan, but while attempting to live on $18 a month, $8 of which went for a room, he acquired pneumonia followed by an unrecognized empyema, which sapped his strength and prevented him from continuing his undergraduate studies. He later entered New York University, from which he received his medical degree in 1888. He spent a year in Germany studying neurology, and after his return to New York was appointed instructor in nervous and mental diseases under Dana at the New York Post-Graduate Hospital Medical School. When Dana transferred to the Bellevue Hospital Medical College, Collins succeeded him at the Post-Graduate Hospital Medical School, holding the title of professor of diseases of the mind and nervous system. During his tenure there he translated into English Jakob's *Atlas of the Normal and Pathological Nervous Systems* (62). He also worked with E. Onufrowicz at the newly established Pathological Institute of the New York State Hospitals on Ward's Island, and with him published an extensive monograph, "Experimental Researches on the Sympathetic Nervous System" in 1900 (32). His book *Treatment of Diseases of the Nervous System* (20) also appeared that year. He held his appointment at the Post-Graduate Hospital Medical School from 1898 to 1909, when he, Fraenkel, and Bailey founded the Neurological Institute of New York. Thereafter he devoted so much of his time and energy to the Institute that it was often referred to as "Dr. Collins' hospital." He also, however, continued to publish scientific articles until 1923, when, with Hideyo Noguchi, he reported on a detailed experimental investigation of the so-called spirochetal etiology of multiple sclerosis which had been proposed by Kuhn and Steiner in 1917 (31). Although he continued to hold his clinical appointment as consulting neurologist at the Neurological Institute of New York, after that date he limited his practice to diagnosis and consulting. Collins was a facile

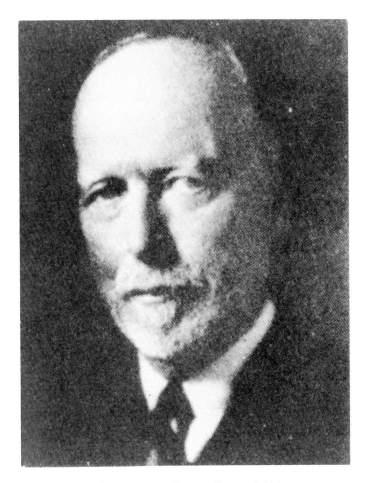

FIG. 19. Joseph Collins. (From ref. 43.)

speaker and writer, and had unlimited energy and working power. He published more than 100 papers as well as medical texts and books of a more literary character. His *Genesis and Dissolution of the Faculty of Speech* (19), a thorough study of aphasia, won for him the Alvarenga Prize of the College of Physicians of Philadelphia. This was followed by *Diseases of the Brain*, *Pathology of the Nervous System*, *The Sympathetic Nervous System*, *Letters to a Neurologist* (21), *The Way with Nerves* (22), and *Sleep and the Sleepless*, all published between 1899 and 1912.

During World War I Collins served in the United States Army in France, first as a major and then as a colonel. After the war he served for a year as director of the American Red Cross in Italy. He was president of the American Neurological Association in 1902.

Collins was a master linguist and wrote critical reviews of French literary figures. His sojourn in Italy gave rise to two appreciative volumes on Italian culture: *My Italian Year* and *Idling in Italy*. Starting in 1923 he published a series of popular books, the best known of which are *The Doctor Looks at Literature* (23), *Taking the Literary Pulse* (24), *The Doctor Looks at Love and Life* (25), *A Doctor Looks at Doctors* (26), *The Doctor Looks at Marriage and Medicine* (27), *The Doctor Looks at Life and Death* (28). A synthesis of his views on medicine appeared in *Some Aspects of the Art and Practice of Medicine* (29). He also wrote a number of articles on medical education and organization which accurately anticipated subsequent development in socialized medicine and group practice. These he incorporated in *The Future of Medicine* (30). He made pleas for liberal social changes, including toleration of sexual deviation, abolition of prohibition, and free dissemination of information on birth control and health education.

Joseph Fraenkel was born in Russia and received his medical education in Vienna. He came to the United States penniless and without friends. He received an appointment as resident physician at the Montefiore Home and Hospital for Chronic Invalids in New York City. Fraenkel spent many hours each day in the hospital studying patients with diseases of the nervous system and soon made an enviable reputation for himself as a neurologist. He worked in dispensaries with Collins, who found him to have excellent clinical insight and judgment. By virtue of his intellectual honesty, kindliness, and industry, he built up a commanding practice with wealthy members of the community within a short time. Fraenkel, along with Collins and Bailey, was a founder of the Neurological Institute of New York, although after only a little more than a year he resigned from its staff. His interests later turned to endocrinology. His publications were few and, except for his role in establishing the Neurological Institute, his influence on neurology was negligible.

Frederick Peterson (1859–1938), (Fig. 20) was born in Fairbault, Minnesota, and was educated in public schools and by private tutors (96), following which he went to the University of Göttingen. He had already decided on a medical career, however, so he returned to the United States and enrolled in the University of Buffalo, from which he received his medical degree in 1879. His special interests were pathology and diseases of the nervous system, and he spent the 3 years following graduation pursuing studies in these fields in Vienna, Zurich, and Strasbourg. On his return to the United States he was appointed professor of pathology at the University of Buffalo but found the field of pathology less rewarding than working with patients with neurologic and mental disorders. To continue his training in the latter field he accepted an appointment as assistant physician in the Poughkeepsie State Hospital. He then became associated with Bernard Sachs, and with him published a detailed study on the infantile cerebral palsies (80). In 1888 he was appointed chief of the neurology clinic at the

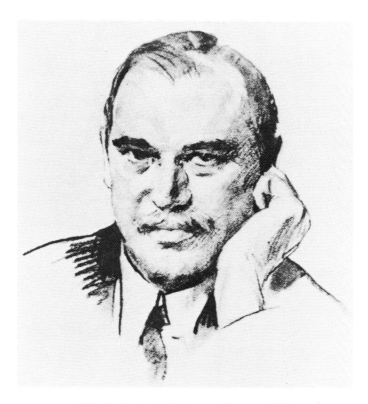

FIG. 20. Frederick Peterson. (From ref. 96.)

College of Physicians and Surgeons of Columbia University under M. Allen Starr.

During the early 1900s Peterson played a major role in guiding neurology and psychiatry to a position of prominence in America. Recognizing the plight of the epileptic patient, for whom little treatment was available at that time, he helped to found the Craig Colony for Epileptics (78). His progressive approach to the problems of the insane led to his appointment as head of the New York State Lunacy Commission. Appalled at the threatened closing of the Neurological Institute of New York by its trustees after Fraenkel's departure in 1911 because of financial difficulties, he joined with Collins, Bailey, and Dana to assume the responsibility for its reorganization and future course. He was instrumental in bringing Adolph Meyer to the New York State Psychiatric Institute, a move that helped shape the development of the Institute as a major research and training center.

Despite his increasing responsibilities, Peterson carried on an active practice in neuropsychiatry, participated in the training of medical students and house staff officers, and made extensive contributions to the scientific literature. His more than 200 publications covered a wide range of neurologic and psychiatric topics. With Archibald Church he published a *Text-Book of Nervous and Mental Disease* that was issued in several editions (18), and with W. S. Haines published a *Text-Book of Legal Medicine and Toxicology* (79). He was a frequent contributor to the popular magazines of the day, including *Collier's Weekly*, *Scriber's Magazine*, and *Atlantic Monthly*. He published a number of collections of poems, and a volume of four original plays. He was a scholarly man, having a profound knowledge of Chinese life and art and a large collection of Chinese treasures. One of his volumes of verse, *Chine Lyrics*, was so faithful to the Chinese imagery and mode of expression that many readers believed it to have been the product of a Chinese writer. He, with Dana, Collins, and Sachs, founded the Charaka Club, and he made many contributions to its literature. Peterson's contributions to his field were well recognized by his contemporaries. He served as Chairman of the Section of Neurology and Medical Jurisprudence of the American Medical Association, president of the New York Neurological Society from 1899 to 1910, and president of the American Neurological Association in 1925.

Charles Albert Elsberg (1871–1948) was one of the twentieth century poineers who helped found a scientific basis for the evolving discipline of neurosurgery (33). He, with Harvey Cushing and Charles Frazier, persuaded the American College of Surgeons to designate neurosurgery a separate specialty. He was graduated from the College of the City of New York and the College of Physicians and Surgeons of Columbia University. His early neurologic associations were with Sachs at Mount Sinai Hospital and Dana at Cornell University, and he did his first clinical and experimental surgery at Mount Sinai Hospital and the Rockefeller Institute. Bailey, Collins, and Fraenkel asked him to join them at the founding of the Neurological Institute of New York, where he was senior attending neurosurgeon from 1910 until 1938. He was the first to occupy the chair of neurosurgery at the College of Physicians, where he served as professor of neurosurgery from 1923 until 1939. His special interest was surgery of the spinal cord and its membranes, and he made significant contributions to this field (47). He was editor of the *Bulletin of the Neurological Institute of New York* from 1932 to 1936 and president of the American Neurological Association in 1938. His last book, *The Story of a Hospital* (46), was the history of the Neurological Institute, during the early development of which he played a significant role.

NEUROLOGY AND PSYCHIATRY DURING THE
FIRST WORLD WAR

The First World War offered an unparalleled opportunity for the various medical specialties to care for the sick and wounded. This was especially true for neurology and psychiatry, which were closely associated at this time (93). It was during this period that the term neuropsychiatry (now no longer in vogue) came into general use. The part that the staff of the Neurological Institute of New York played in the war has already been alluded to. On the day that diplomatic relations with Germany were broken off, Bailey, Stewart Paton, and Thomas Salmon were dining together (46) in New York City discussing the neurologic problems that might arise in case of war. They discussed the very same problems on the following day at a meeting in Washington with Surgeon General Gorgas. The Surgeon General accepted their suggestions, and the three physicians were asked to inspect and report on the neuropsychiatric conditions in army camps in Texas and in the United States Disciplinary Barracks at Fort Leavenworth, Kansas, as well as to assess the facilities for the care of patients with nervous and mental diseases in the event of war.

The National Committee for Mental Hygiene rendered conspicuous service to the United States Army at this time. A special committee on war work was appointed, and Pearce Bailey served as chairman until January 30, 1918, when he was succeeded by Charles L. Dana. The committee faced three problems: a) neurologic and psychiatric evaluation of recruits, b) the treatment of soldiers who developed neurologic or psychiatric problems while in service, and c) continued treatment of such soldiers who were invalided home. The Division of Neurology and Psychiatry, created in the office of the Surgeon General in July 1917 with Bailey in charge, took over the functions that had been performed by the National Committee for Mental Hygiene. The accomplishments of the Division are due largely to Bailey's foresight and organizing ability. After Salmon inspected hospitals in England and observed neuropsychiatric problems there, it became apparent that many more neurologists were needed than were available. Intensive instruction courses in neurology were established at the Neurological Institute of New York under Walter Timme, at the Boston Psychopathic Hospital under E. E. Southard, at the Philadelphia General Hospital under T. H. Weisenburg, at the Phipps Clinic in Baltimore under Adolf Meyer, at St. Elizabeth's Hospital in Washington under William A. White, at the State Psychopathic Hospital in Ann Arbor under Albert M. Barrett, and at Mendocino State Hospital in Talmage, California. Instruction courses in neurosurgery were established in New York under Charles A. Elsberg, in Philadelphia under Charles H. Frazier, in Chicago under Dean Lewis, and in St. Louis under Ernest Sachs.

After troops were sent to Europe in the American Expeditionary Force (A.E.F.) neuropsychiatric units were established in each base hospital. Colonel Harvey Cushing was the senior consultant in the A.E.F., and Lieutenant Colonel Sidney I. Schwab was the medical director of a special base hospital for psychoneuroses at Lafauche. Other consultants at base hospitals were Colonel Daniel J. McCarthy, Major John J. Thomas, Major George E. Price, Major Lewis J. Pollock, Major Andrew H. Woods, and Major J.

Ramsay Hunt. Two hospitals for patients with psychoneuroses and psychoses were established with Lieutenant Colonel Schwab and Lieutenant Colonel Sanger Brown in charge. Neurosurgery in the A.E.F. was under the supervision of Col. Cushing. Toward the end of the war Col. Cushing and Lt. Cols. McCarthy and Schwab formulated a plan whereby the valuable experience obtained in the treatment of neuropsychiatric diseases and injuries during the war could be utilized in the rehabilitation of discharged men. They also prepared a detailed plan for the organization of a central neuropsychiatric institute in Washington and transmitted it to the Surgeon General. The release of ex-servicemen, however, had already started by the time the proposal was reviewed by the Surgeon General; moreover, discharges from the armed forces had become disorganized and were influenced by political pressures, so the plan was never adopted.

MEDICAL AND NEUROLOGIC EDUCATION

The early medical schools were associated with colleges or universities. During the latter years of the nineteenth century and the first part of the twentieth century, however, a large number of private or proprietary schools was established, many with no or inadequate facilities. Early medical education consisted almost entirely of lectures, occasionally accompanied by a patient demonstration. There was no bedside instruction, and the majority of the medical schools had no laboratories and no associated hospital (14,42). Although most of the medical schools taught regular medicine, some taught homeopathic medicine, and there were a few eclectic and naturopathic schools.

Early medical education consisted of 2 years of instruction, although sometimes the second year was a repetition of the same didactic lectures that were given the first year. In 1853 the Chicago Medical College introduced a 3-year graded course. In 1871 Harvard Medical School increased its entrance requirements, increased instruction to 3 years of 9 months each, and graded this course. In 1880 the course was increased to 4 years, and by the turn of the century most of the other medical colleges had done so as well and had added dissection and chemistry laboratories.

In 1909 and 1911 Abraham Flexner conducted extensive studies of the state of medical education in the United Satates and Europe for the Carnegie Foundation for the Advancement of Teaching (48,49). His report contained candid and drastic criticism of the defects in medical education. There were wretched deficiencies in most of the 155 American schools surveyed. The laboratories and clinical facilities were markedly deficient in many of them, and the teaching was often haphazard. Only 14 of the 155 colleges had laboratory facilities for the clinical departments. The report was widely publicized; and many of the colleges, unable to establish laboratories or improve their facilities for clinical instruction, were forced to close. Of the 24 medical colleges in Missouri, only 12 were able to continue; of 43 in New York State, 11 continued; and of 27 in Indiana, 2 remained. Of those that survived, many merged for mutual strengthening, and most secured university affiliation.

Neurology continued to be taught and practiced with psychiatry during this period, but with increasing frequency neurology became a separate section in medical schools with its own faculty (90).

ASSOCIATION FOR RESEARCH IN NERVOUS
AND MENTAL DISEASE

In 1919 Walter Timme, an attending physician at the Neurological Institute of New York, imbued with the spirit of advancing the knowledge of nervous and mental diseases, suggested the formation of the Association for Research in Nervous and Mental Disease (46). This project, to which Timme devoted much of his time and thought, was hailed by his colleagues in the Institute and by neurologists and psychiatrists all over the United States. The founders of this new organization envisaged an entirely new type of medical meeting, one devoted to a single subject chosen several years in advance. Scientists who had done specific basic research on the subject or who had had outstanding clinical experience with it were asked to participate, and the entire proceedings of each annual meeting, along with the complete discussions of the individual's presentation, were to be published in book form. The first meeting was in 1920, and the membership of the Association increased rapidly thereafter, soon including most of the neurologists, pyschiatrists, and neuroscientists in the country who had made significant contributions to their individual fields. The annual meetings, held in New York City close to the Christmas holiday season, were well attended. Dr. Timme served as president for the first few years, after which the members each year elected someone who had made significant contributions to the subject under discussion. The topics discussed during the first 10 annual meetings of the association were as follows: Acute Epidemic Encephalitis (Lethargic Encephalitis); Multicple Sclerosis (Disseminated Sclerosis); Heredity in Nervous and Mental Diseases; The Human Cerebrospinal Fluid; Schizophrenia (Dementia Praecox); The Cerebellum; Epilepsy and the Convulsive State; The Intracranial Pressure on Health and Disease; The Vegetative Nervous System; Manic Depressive Psychosis.

ADVANCES IN NEUROLOGIC DIAGNOSIS AND TREATMENT

More significant advances were made in neurologic diagnosis and treatment than in the basic neurologic sciences during this period.

The X-ray was described by Roentgen in 1895. Lumbar puncture was performed by Corning and others before the turn of the century, and soon the cytologic, chemical, bacteriologic, and serologic examination of the cerebrospinal fluid (CSF) became a part of the routine examination of most patients with diseases of the nervous system. In 1918 Walter E. Dandy of Baltimore performed roentgenography of the brain after injecting air directly into the cerebral ventricles, terming the procedure ventriculography (39). The following year he performed roentgenography of the brain after injecting air into the spinal canal (pneumoencephalography) (40). In 1919 James B. Ayer of Boston and associates described puncture of the cisterna magna for obtaining CSF (rather than puncture of the lumbar spine (4,94)). In 1922 Sicard and Forestier of France described roentgenography of the spinal canal following injection of an iodized medium into the subarachnoid space (myelography) (85). Soon pneumoencephalography and myelography became essential parts of the neurologic appraisal in patients suspected of having specific diseases of the brain or spinal cord, and ventriculography was used in patients suspected of having neurosurgical conditions.

Specific modes of therapy for most diseases of the nervous system were still not available. At the turn of the century bromides were the only drugs known to be of value in the treatment of epilepsy, but their sedative action and frequent side effects made them far from satisfactory. The first hypnotic barbiturate, Veronal (barbital), was introduced in 1883 by Fischer and von Mering. In 1912 Hauptmann demonstrated that phenylethyl barbituric acid (phenobarbital, Luminal) was more effective than other barbiturates, and it soon replaced bromides as the major drug used in the treatment of epilepsy. The first American clinical reports of the use of phenobarbital in epilepsy were those of Dercum (44) in 1919, Grinker (55) in 1920, and Sands (84) in 1921.

Because of the frequency of its occurrence, central nervous system (CNS) syphilis was one of the most important diseases of the nervous system during the early twentieth century. Its two most common manifestations were general paresis (dementia paralytica) and tabes dorsalis. Examination of the CSF was important in its diagnosis. In 1908 the Wassermann test became available for confirmation of the diagnosis, and later other serologic tests such as those described by Kolmer and Kahn came into use. More specific tests have now replaced these. The colloidal gold test was described by Lange in 1912, and other colloidal reactions were also available. Their use was discontinued when more specific and quantitative determinations of the globulins in the CSF came into use. Although these tests aided in the diagnosis of CNS syphilis, treatment (with arsenicals and heavy metals) was far from satisfactory, and specific therapy was not available until the discovery of penicillin and other antibiotics.

During the years just after the First World War there was a widespread pandemic of a hitherto unknown variety of encephalitis—lethargic encephalitis, or von Economo's disease. No specific causal agent was ever demonstrated, and the disease apparently disappeared spontaneously after about 10 years. The mortality rate was quite high, and a majority of patients who survived had serious sequelae. In children these were characterized as behavioral disorders and in adults as a syndrome closely resembling Parkinson's disease, occasionally accompanied by ocular symptoms (oculogyric crises) and respiratory anomalies.

It was during this period that neurosurgery had its birth. A few surgical operations had been performed on the brain and spinal cord in Europe and the United States during the latter part of the nineteenth century, but neurosurgery as a specialty did not exist. In America it evolved from the work of Harvey Cushing in Baltimore and later in Boston, Charles Frazier in Philadelphia, and Charles Elsberg in New York. These three men and their contemporaries, as well as those who trained under them, are largely responsible for the rapid development of neurosurgery in the United States.

Although significant advances were to be made in the basic neurosciences during the first half of the twentieth century, most of the investigations that were started during the first 25 years were not completed until later. This includes the work of Dusser de Barenne, Erlanger and Gasser, Harrison, Huber and Crosby, Larsell, Papez, Ransom, Rasmussen, and others. The principal investigator during this period, and one who made noteworthy contributions, was Cannon.

Walter B. Cannon (1871–1945) (Fig. 21) was born in Prairie du Chien, Wisconsin. It is of interest that this was the site of Fort Crawford, one of the places William Beaumont had studied the gastric digestion of Alexis St. Martin, who had developed a gastric fistula following a gunshot wound of the abdomen (6). After his graduation from Harvard Medical School in 1900, Cannon was appointed instructor in physiology at Harvard, and 6 years later he succeeded Henry P. Bowditch as professor of physiology. In 1896, shortly after he had entered medical school, Cannon demonstrated for the first time, using the newly discovered X-rays, the movements of the alimentary tract. He spent the next few years investigating gastrointestinal physiology, and his studies are summarized in *The Mechanical Factors of Digestion* (10), published in 1911. He ranks with Beaumont and Pavlov as one of the great contributors to our knowledge of the physiology of the digestive tract.

In 1912 the observation that movements of the stomach and intestines ceased when experimental animals were excited stimulated his interest in the new autonomic nervous system, and during the next 20 years he and his students published a number of important papers on the autonomic nervous system and its functions. Some of this work is summarized in his book *Bodily Changes in Pain, Hunger, Fear and Rage* (11), which was published in 1915. The importance of the sympatho-adrenal system in the maintenance of homeostasis, or the stability of the internal environment of the organism, is described in *The Wisdom of the Body* (12). In his autobiography *The Way of an Investigator: A Scientist's Experience in Medical Research* he states

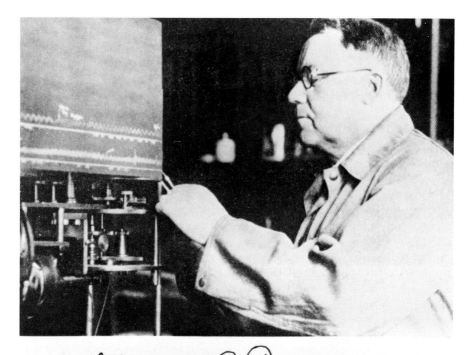

FIG. 21. Walter B. Cannon. (From ref. 6.)

that if he had not undertaken research on the physiology of the digestive tract following his observations with the newly discovered X-rays he would have been a clinical neurologist (13).

PROMINENT AMERICAN NEUROLOGISTS OF THE FIRST QUARTER OF THE TWENTIETH CENTURY

A galaxy of American physicians and neuroscientists played a part in the growth of American neurology during the first quarter of the twentieth century. Those who made the most significant contributions are discussed in some detail.

Smith Ely Jelliffe (1866–1945) (Fig. 22) was born in New York City (7,67). He received a bachelor's degree from the Brooklyn Polytechnic Institute, a medical degree from the College of Physicians and Surgeons of Columbia University, and a doctor of philosophy degree from Columbia University with a thesis on a botanical subject. He had many interests, including botany, pharmacy, pathology, comparative neuroanatomy, embryology, and

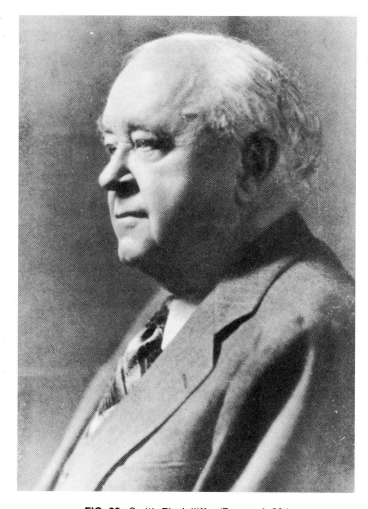

FIG. 22. Smith Ely Jelliffe. (From ref. 66.)

toxicology. In psychiatry he was interested first in the psychoses and later in mental deficiency, hypnosis, the psychoneuroses, and psychotherapy. He had an early interest in psychoanalysis. He was a prodigious writer on many subjects: botany, pharmacy, comparative neuroanatomy, human neuro-anatomy, organic neurologic diseases, psychiatry, psychotherapy, and psychoanalysis. He had a long and creative friendship with William A. White, and with him wrote *Diseases of the Nervous System: A Textbook of Nervous and Mental Disease* (64). He was associate editor of the *Journal of Nervous and Mental Disease* from 1899 to 1902, at which time he purchased the journal and was managing editor from that time until shortly before his death in 1945 (63). He also served as editor of other journals during his long and productive career: associate editor of the *New York Medical Journal* from 1905 to 1909 as well as editor of the *Psychoanalytic Review, Medical News, Transactions of the American Neurological Association,* and the *Journal of Pharmacology.* He was president of the American Neurological Association in 1930. Jelliffe was a large man with enormous energy and had the admiration and affection of the leaders in American neurology and psychiatry as expressed in the numerous tributes to him published in an anniversary number of the *Journal of Nervous and Mental Disease* honoring him in 1935, and again in the obituaries published at the time of his death (68).

James Ramsay Hunt (1874–1937), born in Philadelphia of Quaker parents (70), received a medical degree from the University of Pennsylvania in 1893. During his 2-year internship at the University of Pennsylvania Hospital, Mills stimulated his interest in neurology. He also spent some time at the Episcopal Hospital, where he studied the pathology of paralysis agitant. He presented his first paper on this subject before the Philadelphia Neurological Society in 1895 when he was 21 years of age, and published it in the *Journal of Nervous and Mental Disease* the following year (57). After his internship he spent some time in Europe, studying under Obersteiner in Vienna, Cassirer and Oppenheim in Berlin, and Marie, Dejerine, and Babinski in Paris. He then returned to Philadelphia where he worked in Charles W. Burr's clinic at the Medico-Chirurgical College and continued his study of paralysis agitans.

In 1900 Hunt went to New York where he joined Dana at the Cornell University Medical College as clinical assistant; in 1910 he was made an instructor. He was very active in clinical neurology while at Cornell and made many important contributions. In 1907 he published the first of his papers on herpetic inflammation of the geniculate ganglion, a condition later known as the Ramsay Hunt syndrome (58). Subsequently he conducted several studies of the sensory functions of the seventh nerve.

In 1910 Hunt became associated with the neurology department of the College of Physicians and Surgeons of Columbia University, where he remained until his retirement. Here he went back to the work he had started with Mills in Philadelphia—the clinical and pathologic aspects of the extrapyramidal disorders and also disturbances of cerebellar function. In 1914 his study of dyssynergia cerebellaris progressive was published in *Brain* (59). Later he described another form of the disorder with associated myoclonus, attributing it to atrophy of the dentate nucleus. In his reports on cerebrovascular disease he pointed out that occlusion of the internal carotid artery may produce the same clinical picture as occlusion of the middle cerebral artery and stated that palpation of the internal carotid artery in the neck should be an important part of the physical examination of every stroke patient. He was very much interested in the juvenile form of paralysis agitans, which he attributed to atrophy of the motor cells in globus pallidus (60). His presidential address before the American Neurological Association in 1920 consisted of a review of his studies on the basal ganglia and their disorders (61).

He was a deliberate, meticulous worker, and published his papers after much rewriting. His keen clinical observations brought to light several conditions previously unrecognized. In addition to Hunt's syndrome (geniculate herpes) his name has also been given to neuropathic atrophy of the small muscles of the hand (Hunt's atrophy), dyssynergia cerebellaris myoclonica (Hunt's disease), geniculate neuralgia (Hunt's neuralgia), and atrophy or degeneration of the pallidal system (Hunt's striatal syndrome).

Walter Timme (1874–1956) was born in New York City and graduated from the College of Physicians and Surgeons of Columbia University in 1897. He joined the staff of the Neurological Institute as an assistant physician in 1911, a position he held until he was appointed assistant attending physician in 1915; he later became attending physician (1920) and senior attending physician (1929). He was for many years professor of nervous and mental disease at the New York Polyclinic Hospital and clinical professor of neurology at the College of Physicians and Surgeons. Early in his medical career he became interested in endocrinology, and when an endocrinology service was established at the Neurological Institute in 1934 he was placed in charge of it. During the First World War he was in charge of the courses in neuropsychiatry given at the Institute for army officers. He conceived the idea of the Association for Research in Nervous and Mental Disease, was influential in its formation, and was its president for its first few years.

Frederick Tilney (1876–1938) (Fig. 23) was born in Brooklyn, New York (73). He graduated from Yale University in 1897 and received his medical degree from the Long Island Hospital Medical College in 1903. Following 2 years of study in Berlin he was appointed an assistant in neuroanatomy under George S. Huntington at the College of Physicians and Surgeons, and received a Ph.D. degree in 1912. He became assistant professor of neurology at the College of Physicians and Surgeons in 1914, and the following year he succeeded Starr as professor of neurology. He was actively interested in neuroanatomy and clinical neurology, and authored many important publications. In 1920 he and Henry A. Riley published *The Form and Functions of the Central Nervous System* (91), which in itself was a remarkable contribution to neurology. His interest in the encephalitis epidemic that started in 1917 resulted in his publishing the book *Epidemic Encephalitis*, also in 1920, and led to an appointment to the Matheson Commission, which was established to study epidemic encephalitis and its sequelae. He was attending physician at the Neurological Institute from 1920 to 1930, senior attending physician from 1930 to 1935, and medical director from 1935 to 1938. He was president of the American Neurological Association in 1926.

Edwin Garvin Zabriskie (1874–1959), born in Brooklyn, New York, was graduated from the Long Island Hospital Medical College in 1897 (71). After

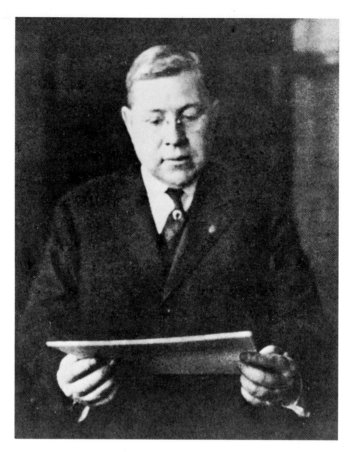

FIG. 23. Frederick Tilney. (From ref. 43.)

study in Paris and Berlin, he entered the practice of neuropsychiatry in New York City. He joined the staff of the Neurological Institute of New York in 1910, was a leading figure in its early years, played an important role in transferring it to the Columbia-Presbyterian Medical Center, and was acting director from 1946 to 1948. He was professor of clinical neurology at the College of Physicians and Surgeons of Columbia University for many years. A founding member of the American Board of Psychiatry and Neurology and of the Association for Research in Nervous and Mental Disease, Zabriskie was president of the American Neurological Association in 1944. He was a consultant in neuropsychiatry to the American Expeditionary Forces during the First World War and was thereafter affectionately known as the "Colonel" by his friends and colleagues. His publications dealt mainly with clinical analysis of diseases of the nervous system. He was director of the laboratories at the Neurological Institute (1911–1916), assistant attending physician (1915–1919), attending physician (1920–1928), senior attending physician (1929–1938), and chief of staff (1935–1938).

Robert Foster Kennedy (1884–1952) was born in Belfast, Ireland, and received his medical degree from the Royal University of Ireland in 1906 (54). Shortly thereafter he was appointed house officer at the National Hospital, Queen Square, London, where he remained for 4 years. In 1910 he came to New York City at the request of Pearce Bailey and joined the staff at the Neurological Institute, and in 1915 was appointed attending physician in the neurology department of Bellevue Hospital and professor of neurology at Cornell University Medical College, positions he held until his retirement. He published more than 200 papers on a variety of neurologic and psychiatric subjects. The syndrome of contralateral papilledema with ipsilateral optic atrophy occurring in association with space-occupying lesions of the frontal lobe is known as the Foster Kennedy syndrome. He was assistant attending physician (1914–1920), attending physician (1920–1934), and consultant in neurology (1934–1938) at the Neurological Institute. His wit, humor, and ability as a raconteur, enhanced by his Irish brogue, made him a favorite teacher and speaker at medical meetings.

William Gibson Spiller (1863–1940) (Fig. 24) was born in Baltimore and in 1892 graduated from the University of Pennsylvania School of Medicine (1,77). He then spent 4 years studying anatomy and pathology under Edinger, Dejerine, and Obersteiner, and clinical neurology under Oppenheim and Gowers. On his return to Philadelphia, he became associated with Mills in clinical neurology and established a laboratory for neuropathology in the Hospital of the University of Pennsylvania. His neuropathologic studies were carried out meticulously. His first clinical work was with Mills at the Philadelphia Polyclinic Hospital, where he was made head of the department of neurology in 1901. He became clinical professor of nervous diseases at the Woman's Medical College of Pennsylvania in 1902, and in 1903 he was made professor of neuropathology and associate professor of neurology at the University of Pennsylvania. On Mills' retirement in 1915, Spiller was made professor of neurology there, a position he held until his own retirement in 1932. In 1935 he was given the honorary degree of Doctor of Science by the University of Pennsylvania.

Spiller made many contributions to neurology, among the more important of which were an accurate delineation of the syndrome of anterior spinal artery occlusion and studies on conjugate ocular movements and internuclear ophthalmoplegia (86). He was interested in problems of pain and conducted detailed studies of the spinothalamic tracts and localization within them. He was the first to recommend spinothalamic tract section for relief of intractable pain in the lower portions of the body (87). He worked with Charles Frazier on the treatment of trigeminal neuralgia, recommending differential section of the nerve to avoid cutting the first division fibers (88). He was appointed associate editor of the *Journal of Nervous and Mental*

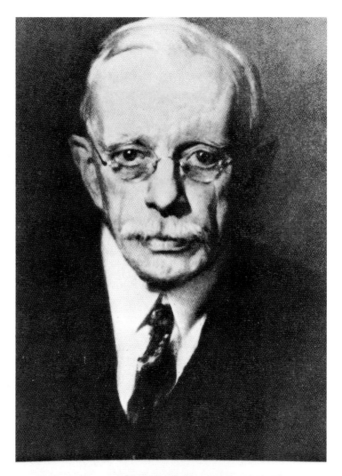

FIG. 24. William G. Spiller. (From ref. 77.)

Disease in 1897 and 2 years later was made editor, serving as editor-in-chief from 1902 to 1913. He was president of the American Neuological Association in 1905. Spiller was a shy, retiring, modest man who gave the impression of being cold and distant, but once his defenses were down he was warm and friendly.

Theodore M. Weisenburg (1875–1934), born in New York City, graduated from the University of Pennsylvania School of Medicine in 1899 (2). He interned in the Philadelphia General Hospital and served for 2 years as an assistant surgeon in the United States Army in the Philippines, and then started the practice of general medicine in Philadelphia. After 18 months he began the study of neurology, to which he devoted the rest of his life. He worked on the wards of the Philadelphia General Hospital with Mills, Spiller, Dercum, and others. He was instructor in neurology and neuropathology in the University of Pennsylvania (1903–1907) and professor of neurology at the Medico-Chirurgical College of Pennsylvania (1907–1915). In 1917 he was appointed professor of neurology in the Graduate School of Medicine of the University of Pennsylvania, a position he held until his death in 1934. He made many contributions to neurology. His fields of major interest were the cerebellum and aphasia, and he was particularly interested in localization within the cerebellum. For about 3 years before his death he was involved in detailed study of aphasia (95). He was president of the American Neurological Association in 1918 and of the Association for Research in Nervous and Mental Disease in 1933. His greatest influence on American neurology was through his position as editor-in-chief of the *Archives of Neurology and Psychiatry*. He was appointed to the editorial board at the time of the establishment of the journal in 1919 and was editor-in-chief from 1920 until his death in 1934.

Charles Harrison Frazier (1870–1936) was born and educated in Philadelphia (56,67). He received his bachelor of arts degree from the University of Pennsylvania in 1889, and not yet having decided on a career he entered the University of Pennsylvania Medical School for 1 year. He remained there, however, and graduated in 1893. He interned in the Episcopal Hospital of Philadelphia and then spent a year in Berlin working under Rudolf Virchow and Ernst von Bergmann. Returning to Philadelphia, he was appointed to the surgical service of the University Hospital and made instructor in clinical surgery in the medical school. In 1901 he was appointed professor of clinical surgery. Frazier's interest in neurosurgery had been stimulated by von Bergmann, and this interest was strengthened in Philadelphia by his association with Mitchell, Mills, Weisenburg, and his classmate Spiller.

In 1919, influenced by his experience with peripheral nerve injuries in France, he decided to devote his work exclusively to neurosurgery. In 1900 and 1901, following the suggestion of Spiller, he showed that the pain of trigeminal neuralgia in the human could be relieved by subtotal retrogasserian neurotomy, with motor function undisturbed and without the development of keratitis sicca (52). In 1905 he, Mills, Weisenburg, and de Schweinitz reported on the surgical removal of tumors of the cerebellum, citing six cases with five recoveries, an unusual report at that time. In 1920 he reported on 500 cases of peripheral nerve injury that had undergone surgery (51). At Spiller's suggestion, Martin had performed the first anterolateral cordotomy for the relief of intactable pain in 1911, but Frazier devised a more practicable operative technique, placing cordotomy among the routine neurosurgical procedures (50).

In 1922 Frazier was made Rhea Barton Professor of Surgery and chairman of the department of surgery at the University of Pennsylvania Medical School. In 1924 the University awarded him the honorary degree of Doctor of Science. He was a founder-member and president of the Society of Neurological Surgeons, and was president of the American Neurological Association in 1929. He, with Cushing and Elsberg, were responsible for the development of neurosurgery in the United States, and many of his trainees went on to develop neurosurgical services and training programs elsewhere, including Alfred Adson at the Mayo Clinic, James Gardner at Western Reserve University, Donald Munro at Harvard University, Max Peet at the University of Michigan, and his successor, Francis Grant, at the University of Pennsylvania.

Frazier was a tall, striking, aristocratic looking man, and a fluent speaker and writer. He was a tireless worker and expected his students and associates to be the same. He would not tolerate argument without fact, and consequently often seemed abrupt and curt. However, those who knew him well found him to be kind and friendly.

Adolf Meyer (1866–1950) was a neuroanatomist, neuropathologist, neurologist, and psychiatrist (82). Born in Switzerland, he studied under August Forel, for whom he wrote a thesis dealing with comparative neuroanatomy. He received his medical degree from the University of Zurich in 1892. He then migrated to America, with no specific position in mind. He entered private practice in Chicago and was appointed docent in neurology (without salary) at the University of Chicago, where he taught an elective course in comparative neuroanatomy. In May 1893 he accepted a position as pathologist at the Eastern State Hospital in Kankakee, Illinois, where he remained for 2.5 years. Here he found that the physicians had no knowledge of either neurology or psychiatry, the psychiatric diagnoses were haphazard, and there was no treatment beyond custodial care. He initiated courses in neuroanatomy and psychiatry for the staff and made efforts to improve patient care. It was at this time that he began to develop his psychiatric philosophy of studying the ''whole man,'' including the patient's life history, his mental status, his family and social setting, as well as his brain (75).

In November 1885 Meyer accepted the position of pathologist and director of clinical laboratory work at the Worcester (Massachusetts) Insane Hospital and docent in psychiatry at Clark University. In 1902 he became director of the Pathological (psychiatric) Institute of the New York State Hospitals and professor of psychiatry at Cornell University Medical College. Each move gave him increased facilities for clinical investigation, research, and teaching. In 1909 he became professor of psychiatry and director of the

Henry Phipps Psychiatric Clinic at the Johns Hopkins Medical School, positions he held until his retirement (45). He is known principally as a psychiatrist, but he also made important contributions to neuroanatomy (83) and neurology. He was president of the American Neurological Association in 1922 and of the American Psychiatric Association in 1927 (74).

Harvey Williams Cushing (1869–1932) (Fig. 25) was born in Cleveland, Ohio (3,8,53). Known generally as Harvey Cushing, he was not the "father" of neurosurgery, an honor that should probably go to Victor Horsley. Cushing, however, revived interest in the specialty and nurtured it by demonstrating that with skilled surgical techniques operations on the nervous system could be carried out safely and with a very low mortality rate. Cushing was graduated from Yale College in 1891 and from Harvard Medical School in 1895, and then spent a year as a surgical house officer at the Massachusetts General Hospital. In 1896 he became assistant resident to William S. Halstead at the Johns Hopkins Hospital, under whom he developed his surgical skills. It was at Johns Hopkins, also, that he developed close friendships with William Osler and William Henry Welch. In June 1900 he went to Europe for 14 months. In Switzerland he worked under Theodore Kocher, whose book on spinal cord injuries interested him, and in the laboratory of the physiologist Hugo Kronecker, where his study of the CSF led him eventually to his analysis of the effects of increased intracranial pressure on the blood pressure, pulse, and respiration. He was stimulated to delve more deeply into neurophysiology by Charles Sherrington, who was then in Liverpool.

He returned to The Johns Hopkins Hospital and began his career as a neurosurgeon. In 1912 he was appointed Moseley Professor of Surgery at Harvard Medical School and Surgeon-in-Chief at the Peter Bent Brigham Hospital. During the First World War he was in charge of neurosurgery with the American Expeditionary Forces in France, after which he returned to Harvard and the Peter Bent Brigham Hospital. On his retirement in 1932 he was appointed Sterling Professor of Neurology at Yale University and Director of Studies in the History of Medicine.

Cushing perfected neurosurgery. He developed technical procedures that minimized hemorrhage during all operations that involved the brain and spinal cord. His international fame as a neurosurgeon started in 1910 when he was called on to remove a large meningioma from Major General Leonard Wood, Chief of Staff of the United States Army. The operation was successful, and General Wood returned to his official duties within a month, served throughout World War I, and later was appointed Governor General of the Philippine Islands. Cushing was also known as a teacher of neurosurgeons, and those who trained under him include Walter Dandy of Johns Hopkins Medical School, Percival Bailey of the University of Chicago, Jason Mixter of Harvard Medical School, Gilbert Horrax of Boston, Howard Naffziger of San Francisco, Carl Rand of Los Angeles, Kenneth McKenzie

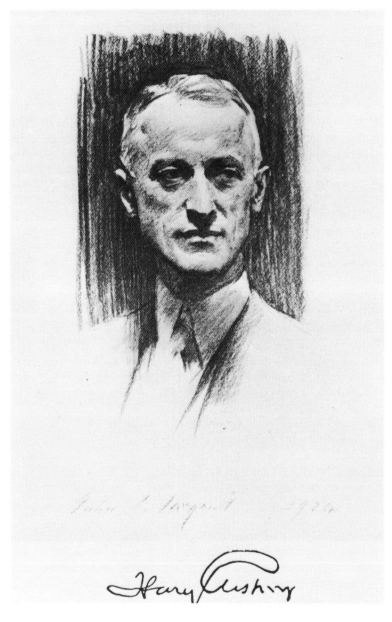

FIG. 25. Harvey Cushing. (From ref. 53.)

of Toronto, Norman Dott of Edinburgh, Geoffrey Jefferson and Hugh Cairns of England, and many others.

Cushing was a prolific writer, and his bibliography has been published in book form. His published works were models of medical writing, each having been rewritten many times, to the exasperation of his secretaries. Among the more important of his books are as follows: *The Pituitary Body and Its Disorders* (34), *Tumors of the Nervus Acousticus and Syndromes of the Cerebellopontile Angle* (35), *A Classification of the Tumors of the Glioma Group on a Histogenetic Basis, with a Correlated Study of Prognosis* (with Percival Bailey), *Intracranial Tumors* (37), and *Meningiomas* (the latter two with Louise Eisenhardt (38)). He was also a student of the history of medicine and had an immense library of important books on the subject, which he left to Yale University. One of his important achievements outside of the field of neurosurgery was his detailed, personal, two-volume *The Life of Sir William Osler* (36), which won him a Pulitzer Prize. Cushing was president of the American Neurological Association in 1923. To honor him, his friends and former pupils formed the Harvey Cushing Society, later to be known as the American Association of Neurological Surgeons.

Walter Edward Dandy (1886–1946) did much to improve the techniques of neurosurgery (92). Born in Sedalia, Missouri, he graduated from the University of Missouri, after which he entered The Johns Hopkins Medical School, from which he was graduated in 1910. He stayed on as a house officer at The Johns Hospital and then began his career as an investigator, innovative neurosurgeon, and prolific writer. His early important articles on the production and absorption of CSF and the pathogenesis of hydrocephalus were written in collaboration with Blackfan. What may have been his greatest contributions to neurosurgery were his introduction of ventriculography in 1918 and of pneumoencephalography the following year (39,40).

Following these experimental studies, Dandy's interests turned more and more toward the development and perfection of neurosurgical techniques. In 1926 he described a posterior approach to the section of the trigeminal root in the treatment of trigeminal neuralgia. This procedure proved to be easier, simpler, safer, and less apt to be complicated by keratitis and facial weakness than the retrogasserian neurectomy described by Spiller and Frazier. He devised a differential section of the vestibular portion of the eighth nerve for the treatment of Meniere's syndrome. He showed that cerebral aneurysms were amenable to surgical treatment and wrote an important monograph on the subject (41). Although not one of the pioneer neurosurgeons, he did much to advance the specialty.

Hugh Talbot Patrick (1860–1939) was born in New Philadelphia, Ohio (43,65,69). He attended Wooster (Ohio) College and the Bellevue Hospital Medical College, from which he graduated in 1884. He entered the practice of neurology and psychiatry in Chicago in 1886, being the first Chicago neurologist to enter the field without serving in a state hospital first. Instead, he did postgraduate work in Germany, France, and England, where he made many friends with whom he corresponded throughout his life, and for whom he became the only known neurologist in the American Middle West. In 1891 he was appointed professor of nervous and mental disease at the Chicago Polyclinic and in 1895 instructor in nervous and mental diseases at the Northwestern University Medical School, rising to the rank of professor in 1902 and professor emeritus in 1919. He was one of the founders of the *Archives of Neurology and Psychiatry* and served on the editorial board during its first few years; for many years he was also editor of the *Yearbook of Neurology and Psychiatry*. Patrick was one of the founders of the Chicago Neurological Society, its first secretary, and twice its president. He was president of the American Neurological Association in 1907. His voluminous bibliography shows a wide range of neurologic interests. It is said that he brought scientific neurology to Chicago.

  Peter Bassoe (1873–1945) was born in Drammen, Norway, and came to the United States at the age of 19 (9,69). He taught in a country school in Iowa, but his interest soon turned to medicine and he graduated from the College of Medicine of the University of Illinois in 1897. Following a year of internship at the Cook County Hospital, he became assistant physician at the State Hospital for the Insane in Mt. Pleasant, Iowa. After 2 years he transferred to the Massachusetts State Hospital at Worcester to work with Adolph Meyer who had just arrived there. In 1901 he went to Europe to study at Heidelberg, Montpelier, and Prague. In 1902 he returned to Chicago to work with Thor C. Rothstein in neuropathology but in 1906 went to Europe for further study in Berlin, Paris, and London. In 1907 he again returned to Chicago and became associated with Hugh T. Patrick. Bassoe was appointed attending neurologist at the Cook County Hospital and assistant professor of nervous diseases at the Rush Medical College, where he was later promoted to the rank of professor and made chairman of the department. He assisted Patrick in editing the *Year Book of Neurology and Psychiatry* from 1910 to 1918, and was sole editor from 1918 until 1933. He published more than 100 papers on a wide range of neurologic subjects and was highly regarded as a teacher. His familiarity with the neurologic literature was extensive. He became a member of the American Neurological Association in 1911 and was its president in 1927. He believed, however, that the membership of the Association was too small and that it was dominated by neurologists from the eastern seaboard. As a consequence he planned and founded the Central Neuropsychiatric Association and was its first president.

  Charles Gilbert Chaddock (1861–1935) was born in Jonesville, Michigan, the son of a physician (76). He graduated from the Department of Medicine and Surgery of the University of Michigan in 1885, following which he served as a staff physician at the Northern Michigan Asylum at Traverse

City. He spent the year 1888 to 1889 studying in Europe and on his return to Traverse City was appointed assistant superintendent of the Asylum (later the Traverse City State Hospital). In 1892 he moved to St. Louis, Missouri, where he was appointed professor of nervous and mental diseases at the Marion-Sims Medical College, succeeding Charles H. Hughes. Marion-Sims Medical College later joined the Beaumont Medical College to become the medical department of St. Louis University. The years 1897 to 1899 were spent in Paris as assistant to Joseph Babinski. In later years he returned to Paris frequently, and made long visits there the summers of 1902, 1903, 1908, 1909, 1913, and 1921.

Chaddock's earliest contributions to the medical literature were his translations, mainly on psychiatric subjects. These include his translation of Krafft-Ebing's *Psychopathia Sexualis* in 1892, Schrenk-Notzing's *Therapeutic Suggestion in Psychopathis Sexualis* in 1895, and Krafft-Ebing's *Textbook of Insanity* in 1904. His interests later turned more to neurology, possibly in part due to his close friendship with Babinski. He is best known for his description of the external malleolar sign, generally known as the Chaddock sign, first published in 1911 (15,16). He also described a wrist reflex which is sometimes given his name (17).

REFERENCES

1. Alpers, B. J. (1975): William Gibson Spiller 1863–1930. In: *Centennial Anniversary Volume of the American Neurological Association 1875–1975*, edited by D. Denny-Brown, A. S. Rose, and A. L. Sahs, pp. 122–126. Springer, New York.
2. Alpers, B. J. (1975): Theodore Weisenburg 1876–1934. In: *Centennial Anniversary Volume of the American Neuological Association 1875–1975*, edited by D. Denny-Brown, A. S. Rose, and A. L. Sahs, pp. 142–146. Springer, New York.
3. Anderson, E., and Haymaker, W. (1970): Harvey Cushing (1869–1939). In: *The Founders of Neurology*, 2nd Ed., edited by W. Haymaker and F. Schiller, pp. 543–549. Charles C Thomas, Springfield, Illinois.
4. Ayer, J. B. (1920): Puncture of cisterna magna. *Arch. Neurol. Psychiatry*, 4:529–541.
5. Bailey, P., Jr. (1975): Pearce Bailey 1865–1922. In: *Centennial Anniversary Volume of the American Neurological Association 1875–1975*, edited by D. Denny-Brown, A. S. Rose, and A. L. Sahs, pp. 136–137. Springer, New York.
6. Bard, P. (1970): Walter Cannon (1871–1945). In: *The Founders of Neurology*, 2nd Ed., edited by W. Haymaker and F. Schiller, pp. 279–281. Charles C Thomas, Springfield, Illinois.
7. Brill, A. A. (1947): In memorium: Smith Ely Jelliffe. *J. Nerv. Ment. Dis.*, 106:221–227.
8. Bucy, P. C. (1975): Harvey Cushing 1859–1939. In: *Centennial Anniversary Volume of the American Neurological Association 1875–1975*, edited by D. Denny-Brown, A. S. Rose, and A. L. Sahs, pp. 159–163. Springer, New York.
9. Bucy, P. C. (1975): Petter Bassoe 1874–1943. In: *Centennial Anniversary Volume of the American Neurological Association 1875–1975*, edited by D. Denny-Brown, A. S. Rose, and A. L. Sahs, pp. 174–177. Springer, New York.
10. Cannon, W. B. (1911): *The Mechanical Factors of Digestion*. Longmans, Green & Co., New York.
11. Cannon, W. B. (1915): *Bodily Changes in Pain, Hunger, Fear and Rage*. Appleton, New York.
12. Cannon, W. B. (1932): *The Wisdom of the Body*. Norton, New York.

13. Cannon, W. B. (1845): *The Way of an Investigator: A Scientist's Experience in Medical Research*. Norton, New York.
14. Casamajor, L. (1943): Notes for an intimate history of neurology and psychiatry in America. *J. Nerv. Ment. Dis.*, 98:600–608.
15. Chaddock, C. G. (1911): A preliminary consideration concerning a new diagnostic nervous sign. *Interstate Med. J.*, 12:742–746.
16. Chaddock, C. G. (1911): The external malleolar sign. *Interstate Med. J.*, 13:1026–1038.
17. Chaddock, C. G. (1912): A new reflex phenomenon in the hand: The wrist-sign. *Interstate Med. J.*, 19:127–131.
18. Church, A., and Peterson, F (1899): *Text-Book of Nervous and Mental Diseases*. Philadelphia, Saunders.
19. Collins, J. (1898): *The Genesis and Dissolution of the Faculty of Speech*. Macmillan, New York.
20. Collins, J. (1900): *The Treatment of Diseases of the Nervous System: A Manual for Practitioners*. William Wood and Co., New York.
21. Collins, J. (1908): *Letters to a Neurologist*. William Wood and Co., New York.
22. Collins, J. (1911): *The Way with Nerves*. Putnam, New York.
23. Collins, J. (1923): *The Doctor Looks at Literature*. G. H. Doran Co., New York.
24. Collins, J. (1924): *Taking the Literary Pulse*. G. H. Doran Co., New York.
25. Collins, J. (1926): *The Doctor Looks at Love and Life*. Harper and Brothers, New York.
26. Collins, J. (1927): *A Doctor Looks at Doctors*. Harper and Brothers, New York.
27. Collins, J. (1929): *The Doctor Looks at Marriage and Medicine*. Harper and Brothers, New York.
28. Collins, J. (1931): *The Doctor Looks at Life and Death*. Harper and Brothers, New York.
29. Collins, J. (1933): *Some Aspects of the Art and Practice of Medicine*. University of Kansas Press, Lawrence, Kansas.
30. Collins, J. (1932): The future of medicine. *Psychiat. Q.*, 6:403–416.
31. Collins, J., and Noguchi, H. (1923): An experimental study of multiple sclerosis. *J.A.M.A.*, 81:2109–2112.
32. Collins, J., and Onufrowicz, B. (1900): Experimental research on the sympathetic nervous system. *Arch. Neurol. Psychopathol.*, 3:1–252.
33. Cramer, F. (1975): Charles Albert Elsberg 1871–1948. In: *Centennial Anniversary Volume of the American Neurological Association 1875–1975*, edited by D. Denny-Brown, A. S. Rose, and A. L. Sahs, pp. 211–216. Springer, New York.
34. Cushing, H. (1917): *The Pituitary Body and Its Disorders*. Lippincott, Philadelphia.
35. Cushing, H. (1917): *Tumors of the Nervus Acousticus and Syndromes of the Cerebellopontile Angle*. Saunders, Philadelphia.
36. Cushing, H. (1926): *The Life of Sir William Osler*, 2 vols. Clarendon Press, Oxford.
37. Cushing, H. (1932): *Intracranial Tumors*. Charles C Thomas, Springfield, Illinois.
38. Cushing, H., and Eisenhardt, L. (1938): *Meningiomas*. Charles C Thomas, Springfield, Illinois.
39. Dandy, W. E. (1918): Ventriculography after the injection of air into the cerebral ventricles. *Ann. Surg.*, 55:5–19.
40. Dandy, W. E. (1919): Roentgenography of the brain after the injection of air into the spinal canal. *Ann. Surg.*, 70:397–403.
41. Dandy, W. E. (1944): *Intracranial Arterial Aneurysms*. Comstock Publishing Co., Ithaca, New York.
42. Deitrick, I. C., and Berson, R. C. (1953): *Medical Schools in the United States at Mid-Century*. McGraw-Hill, New York.
43. Denny-Brown, D., Rose, A. S., and Sahs, A. L. (eds.) (1975): *Centennial Anniversary Volume of the American Neurological Association 1875–1975*. Springer, New York.
44. Dercum, F. X. (1919): On the complete control of epileptic seizures by the luminal-technique. *Ther. Gaz.*, 43:609–611.
45. Ebaugh, F. (1951): Adolf Meyer's contribution to psychiatric education. *Johns Hopkins Hosp. Bull.*, 89:73–80.
46. Elsberg, C. A. (1944): *The Story of a Hospital*. Hoeber, New York.
47. Elsberg, C. A. (1916): *The Diagnosis and Treatment of Surgical Diseases of the Spinal Cord and Its Membranes*. Philadelphia, Saunders.

48. Flexner, A. (1912): *Medical Schools in the United States and Canada: A Report to the Carnegie Foundation for the Advancement of Teaching*. New York, Carnegie Foundation.

49. Flexner, A. (1912): *Medical Education in Europe: A Report to the Carnegie Foundation for the Advancement of Teaching*. Carnegie Foundation, New York.

50. Frazier, C. H. (1920): Section of the antero-lateral columns of the spinal cord for the relief of pain. *Arch. Neurol. Psychiatry*, 4:137–147.

51. Frazier, C. H., and Gilbert, S. A. (1920): Observation of five hundred cases of injuries of the peripheral nerves at the U.S.A. General Hospital No. 11. *Surg. Gynecol. Obstet.*, 30:50–63.

52. Frazier, C. H., and Spiller, W. G. (1901): Division of the sensory root of the trigeminus for the relief of tic douloureux: An experimental, pathological study, with a preliminary report of one surgically successful case. *Phila. Med. J.*, 8:1039–1052.

53. Fulton, J. F. (1946): *Harvey Cushing: A Biography*. Charles C Thomas, Springfield, Illinois.

54. Goodell, H., and Plum, F. (1975): *Robert Foster Kennedy 1884–1952*. In: *Centennial Anniversary Volume of the American Neurological Association 1875–1975*, edited by D. Denny-Brown, A. S. Rose, and A. L. Sahs, pp. 220–221. Springer, New York.

55. Grinker, J. (1919): Experiences with luminal in epilepsy. *J.A.M.A.*, 75:88–92.

56. Groff, F. A. (1975): Charles Harrison Frazier 1879–1936. In: *Centennial Anniversary Volume of the American Neurological Association 1875–1975*, edited by D. Denny-Brown, A. S. Rose, and A. L. Sahs, pp. 177–181. Springer, New York.

57. Hunt, J. R. (1896): A contribution to the pathology of paralysis agitans. *J. Nerv. Ment. Dis.*, 23:184–188.

58. Hunt, J. R. (1907): On herpetic inflammation of the geniculate ganglion: A new syndrome and its complications. *J. Nerv. Ment. Dis.*, 34:73–96.

59. Hunt, J. R. (1914): Dyssynergia cerebellaris progressiva: A chronic progressive form of cerebellar tremor. *Brain*, 37:247–268.

60. Hunt, J. R. (1918): Primary atrophy of the pallidal system of the corpus striatum. *Arch. Intern. Med.*, 22:647–691.

61. Hunt, J. R. (1920): The static and kinetic systems of motility. *Arch. Neurol. Psychiatry*, 4:353–368.

62. Jakob, J. (1896): *Atlas of the Normal and Pathological Nervous Systems*, translated by J. Collins. William Wood & Co., New York.

63. Jelliffe, S. E. (1939): The editor himself and his adopted child. *J. Nerv. Ment. Dis.*, 89:545–589.

64. Jelliffe, S. E., and White, W. A. (1915): *Diseases of the Nervous System: A Textbook of Neurology and Psychiatry*. Lea & Febiger, Philadelphia.

65. Kelly, H. A., and Burrage, W. L. (eds.) (1920): *American Medical Biographies*. Norman Remington Company, Baltimore.

66. Kubie, L. S. (1975): Smith Ely Jelliffe 1866–1945. In: *Centennial Anniversary Volume of the American Neurological Association 1875–1975*, edited by D. Denny-Brown, A. S. Rose, and A. L. Sahs, pp. 181–188. Springer, New York.

67. Lewey, F. H. (1970): Charles Harrison Frazier (1870–1936). In: *The Founders of Neurology*, 2nd Ed., edited by W. Haymaker and F. Schiller, pp. 559–562. Charles C Thomas, Springfield, Illinois.

68. Lewis, N. D. C. (1949): Seventy-five years of service. *J. Nerv. Ment. Dis.*, 110:451–463.

69. Mackay, R. P. (1964): The history of neurology in Chicago. *Illinois Med. J.*, 125:51–58, 142–146, 256–259, 341–344, 539–544, 636–640; 126:60–64.

70. McHenry, L. C., Jr. (1975): James Ramsay Hunt 1874–1937. In: *Centennial Anniversary Volume of the American Neurological Association 1875–1975*, edited by D. Denny-Brown, A. S. Rose, and A. L. Sahs, pp. 147–152. Springer, New York.

71. Merritt, H. H. (1975): Edwin Garvin Zabriskie 1874–1959. In: *Centennial Anniversary Volume of the American Neurological Association 1875–1975*, edited by D. Denny-Brown, A. S. Rose, and A. L. Sahs, pp. 239–242. Springer, New York.

72. Mettler, F. A. (1975): Joseph Collins 1866–1950. In: *Centennial Anniversary Volume of the American Neurological Association 1875–1975*, edited by D. Denny-Brown, A. S. Rose, and A. L. Sahs, pp. 117–121. Springer, New York.

73. Mettler, F. A. (1975): Frederick Tilney 1876–1938. In: *Centennial Anniversary Volume of the American Neurological Association 1875–1975*, edited by D. Denny-Brown, A. S. Rose, and A. L. Sahs, pp. 167–174. Springer, New York.

74. Meyer, A. (1928–1929): Twenty-five years of psychiatry in the United States and our present outlook. *Am. J. Psychiatry,* 85:1–31.
75. Meyer, A. (1922): Inter-relations of the domain of neuropsychiatry. *Arch. Neurol. Psychiatry,* 8:111–121.
76. O'Leary, J. L., and Moore, W. L. (1953): Charles Gilbert Chaddock: His life and contributions. *J. Hist. Med. Allied Sci.,* 8:301–317.
77. Ornsteen, A. M. (1975): William Gibson Spiller (1863–1940). In: *The Founders of Neurology,* 2nd Ed., edited by W. Haymaker and F. Schiller, pp. 520–524. Charles C Thomas, Springfield, Illinois.
78. Peterson, F. (1892): Outline of a plan for an epileptic colony. *New York Med. J.,* 56:96–98.
79. Peterson, F., and Haines, W. S. (1920): *Text-Book of Legal Medicine and Toxicology.* Saunders, Philadelphia.
80. Peterson, F., and Sachs, B. (1890): A study of cerebral palsies in early life, based upon an analysis of one hundred and forty cases. *J. Nerv. Ment. Dis.,* 18:295–332.
81. Pool, J. L. (1975): *The Neurological Institute of New York, with Personal Anecdotes.* The Pocket Knife Press, Lakeville, Connecticut.
82. Rioch, D. Mck. (1975): Adolf Meyer 1866–1950. In: *Centennial Anniversary Volume of the American Neurological Association 1875–1975,* edited by D. Denny-Brown, A. S. Rose, and A. L. Sahs, pp. 153–159. Springer, New York.
83. Rose, J. E. (1951): Adolf Meyer's contributions to neuroanatomy. *Johns Hopkins Hosp. Bull.,* 89:56–63.
84. Sands, I. J. (1921): Luminal therapy in the control of epileptic seizures. *Arch. Neurol. Psychiatry,* 5:305–310.
85. Sicard, J. A., and Forestier, J. (1922): Methode generale d'exploration radiologique par l'huile iodée (lipiodal). *Bull. Mem. Soc. Med. Paris,* 45:462–469.
86. Spiller, W. G. (1905): The importance in clinical diagnosis of paralysis of associated movements of the eyeballs, especially of upward and downward associated movements. *J. Nerv. Ment. Dis.,* 32:417–449, 497, 530.
87. Spiller, W. G., and Martin, E. (1912): The treatment of persistent pain of organic origin in the lower part of the body by division of the anterolateral columns of the spinal cord. *J.A.M.A.,* 58:1489–1492.
88. Spiller, W. G., and Frazier, C. H. (1902): The division of the sensory root of the trigeminus for the relief of tic douloureux. *Univ. Penn. Med. Bull.,* 14:342–352.
89. Stookey, B. (1950): Historical background of the Neurological Institute and the neurological societies. *Bull. NY Acad. Med.,* 35:707–729.
90. Stookey, B. (1959): "What is past is prologue." *Arch. Neurol.,* 1:467–474.
91. Tilney, F., and Riley, H. A. (1920): *The Form and Functions of the Central Nervous System.* Hoeber, New York.
92. Walker, A. E.: Walter Dandy (1885–1946). In: *The Founders of Neurology,* 2nd Ed., edited by W. Haymaker and F. Schiller, pp. 548–552. Charles C Thomas, Springfield, Illinois.
93. Weisenburg, T. H. (1924): The military history of the American Neurological Association. In: *Semi-centennial Anniversary Volume of the American Neurological Association,* edited by F. Tilney and S. E. Jelliffe, pp. 262–310. American Neurological Association, New York.
94. Wegeforth, F., Ayer, J. B., and Essick, C. R. (1919): The method of obtaining cerebrospinal fluid by puncture of the cisterna magna (cistern puncture). *Am. J. Med. Sci.,* 157:789–797.
95. Weisenburg, T. H., and McBride, E. E. (1935): *Aphasia: A Clinical and Psychological Study.* The Commonwelath Fund, New York.
96. Yahr, M. D. (1975): Frederick Peterson 1859–1938. In: *Centennial Anniversary Volume of the American Neurological Association 1875–1975,* edited by D. Denny-Brown, A. S. Rose, and A. L. Sahs, pp. 164–167. Springer, New York.

6

American Neurology During the Second Quarter of the Twentieth Century

Several widely separated events, new techniques, and advances in therapy had a major influence on the growth and development of American neurology during the second quarter of the twentieth century. For example, electroencephalography was developed as a diagnostic and research technique, and its utilization spread rapidly. Angiography too was found to be safe and practicable, and became an important diagnostic procedure.

The American Board of Psychiatry and Neurology was established during this period, and to qualify for certification by the Board candidates were required to receive their training in approved programs that adhered to specific standards. During World War II there were increasing demands for neurologists in the armed forces in the United States, the European Theater, and the Far East. Antibiotics were discovered and came into general use, and specific modes of therapy were developed for many disorders of the nervous system. The American Academy of Neurology was organized and grew rapidly. Finally, neurologic and neurosurgical services were opened in many Veterans Administration Hospitals and became important teaching facilities for many medical schools.

ELECTROENCEPHALOGRAPHY

In 1929 Hans Berger, of Jena, first demonstrated the electrical potentials of the brain in man (4). He was not, however, the first person to be aware of their existence (6). In 1875 Richard Caton, in Liverpool, had discovered the intrinsic electrical activity of the brain, noting that when electrodes lay on the cortical surface of the brains of experimental animals there was a continued waxing and waning of potential. This was present in the unstimulated animal and was not related to respiratory or circulatory rhythms. This intrinsic electrical activity of the brain was also found independently 15 years later by Adolph Beck in Poland. It was Berger, however, who demonstrated that brain waves could be recorded in man through the intact skull. He coined the term electroencephalogram and demonstrated that the characteristics of the brain waves could be used as indices of brain disease. He opened new lines of approach to brain mechanisms and disease for the neurophysiologist and clinician.

The discipline of clinical electroencephalography came into its own around 1935, having its major use in the diagnosis and delineation of various types of epilepsy; it is also valuable, however, in the interpretation of localized and generalized brain disease of various types as well as being an important investigative technique. Among the American pioneers in investigative and diagnostic electroencephalography are Robert B. Aird, Cosimo Ajmone-Marsan, Basu K. Bagchi, Reginald G. Bickford, Mary A. G. Brazier, Theodore J. Case, G. E. Chatrian, David D. Daly, Hallowell Davis, Alexander Forbes, Francis M. Forster, Frederic and Erna Gibbs, Gilbert H. Glaser, Eli Goldensohn, Charles E. Henry, Paul F. A. Hoefer, Herbert H. Jasper, Peter Kellaway, John H. Knott, William G. Lennox, Jerome K. Merlis, James L. O'Leary, Robert S. Schwab, and Alphonse R. Vonderaha.

ANGIOGRAPHY

Cerebral angiography was first described by Moniz in 1927 (49), but it was not until the late 1930s and early 1940s that it came into widespread use (47). Because during the early years it was used mainly in the diagnosis of mass lesions of the brain, and because the original carotid artery injections were done by the "cutdown" technique, the procedure was performed largely by neurosurgeons. Later it became apparent that angiography was also of use in the diagnosis of vascular lesions, e.g., aneurysms and intra- and extracranial arterial stenoses and occlusions (21). Using the percutaneous technique, angiography became a widely used diagnostic procedure for neurologists as well as surgeons. Now, with various refinements, it is being taken over by a new subspecialty, neuroradiology.

ADVANCES IN NEUROLOGIC THERAPY

Infectious Diseases

Because of the frequency of its occurrence, central nervous system (CNS) syphilis was one of the most important diseases of the nervous system during the nineteenth century and the early decades of the twentieth century. It manifested most frequently as either general paresis (dementia paralytica) or tabes dorsalis, but the effects of syphilis on the nervous system were legion. In spite of attempts at therapy with arsenicals, heavy metals, and later by artificially induced fever, treatment of CNS syphilis was generally unsuccessful. Penicillin was discovered by Alexander Fleming in 1928 but was relatively neglected for a decade. In 1940 Florey and others developed it as a systemic therapeutic agent, but it was not available for general use until the end of World War II, in 1945. Subsequently the use of it and other antibiotics has almost completely eradicated CNS syphilis (50).

Treatment of the acute bacterial meningitides has always been a major problem for neurologists. The sulfonamides, really our first antibacterial agents, were introduced during the late 1930s. After penicillin was released for general use, other important antibiotics became available. The use of these various agents has significantly reduced the mortality rate and sequelae of these meningitides, and streptomycin, used alone or with other drugs, has reduced the mortality rate and the morbidity of tuberculous meningitis.

Viral diseases of the nervous system are still enigmas as far as treatment is concerned. There is little to offer in the way of specific therapy for most of the viral meningitides and encephalitides. Fortunately, however, most of those encountered today are mild in degree and self-limited in course.

One of the most significant advances in medicine during recent years is the development of a vaccine against poliomyelitis. This viral disease of the nervous system was once a very important cause of death, especially in children, and an even more significant crippling disability starting in early life; it is now almost nonexistent. Research was stimulated, organized, and partially financed by a commission set up by associates and friends of President Franklin D. Roosevelt, himself a victim of the disease. The first poliomyelitis vaccine in general use, an injectable substance that contained killed organisms, was introduced by Jonas Salk in 1955 (65). This has now been largely replaced by an orally administered, attenuated live-virus vaccine introduced by Albert Sabin a few years later (63).

Epilepsy

While clinical electroencephalography, which contributed immeasurably to the study of epilepsy, was being developed, other clinical, pathologic, biochemical, and related studies on epilepsy were also under way, including a search for newer and more effective drugs. H. Houston Merritt and Tracy J. Putnam, in the laboratories of the Boston City Hospital, carried out their investigations by testing the ability of many chemical substances to suppress electroshock convulsions in experimental animals. After testing a number of drugs, they found in 1938 that sodium diphenylhydantoinate (Dilantin, phenytoin) was the most effective. This was a signal advance in antiepileptic therapy because of the drug's efficacy and because it does not have the sedative and depressant action of the drugs then in use (the bromides and phenobarbital). Phenytoin soon became the standard drug for the treatment of major seizures. The development of drugs for treatment of petit mal (absence) attacks was a more difficult problem. Trimethadione (Tridione) and related drugs were introduced in 1944 and shortly thereafter (22). These were not very effective, however, and dangerous side effects were associated with their use. More effective drugs for all types of epilepsy were to become available later.

Neurologists have always worked closely with neurosurgeons, and during the same period that anticonvulsants were being developed advances were being made in the surgical treatment of epilepsy. Surgery had been used prior to this time for the removal of brain tumors and abscesses whose major symptoms had been convulsions, but it was not until the close of the third decade of the century that some neurosurgeons started operative treatment of focal seizures derived from etiologies other than tumor and abscess.

The pioneer in this field in the United States was Wilder Penfield, who had been trained in neurophysiology under Sherrington at Oxford, in neurology under Holmes in London, and in neurosurgery under Foerster in Breslau (5,53). Penfield was born in Spokane, Washington, and did his first epilepsy surgery in New York City at the Presbyterian Hospital and the College of Physicians and Surgeons. He went to Montreal in 1928 as first director of the Montreal Neurological Institute, where surgery of epilepsy became his major investigative and therapeutic endeavor. His approach to such surgery was greatly furthered when Herbert Jasper joined him in 1936 and established the neurophysiology laboratory at the Institute, and it was enhanced even more with the development of electrocorticography, which provides even more precise diagnosis and localization of malfunctioning brain tissue. Interest in the surgical treatment of epilepsy was additionally stimulated after the demonstration, by Jasper and Kershman in 1941, of sharp waves in the temporal areas of the brain in cases of so-called psychomotor epilepsy. They attributed these, as well as the ictal symptoms, to a neuronal discharge located in the temporal lobe and underlying structures. It was found that surgical removal of this discharging focus in many cases resulted in improvement in or cessation of seizures (55).

Vascular Disease

Because of their frequency, the vascular diseases affecting the nervous system have long constituted one of the most important groups of neurologic diseases. Many advances in our knowledge and treatment of them were made during the second quarter of the twentieth century. Sir Charles Symonds had pointed out as early as 1923 that the presence of intracranial aneurysms could be diagnosed during life, and that rupture of such an aneurysm might be one of the causes of spontaneous subarachnoid hemorrhage (70). It took a decade for physicians to appreciate the fact that rupture of an intracranial aneurysm was by far the most important cause of subarachnoid hemorrhage. The advent of arteriography has allowed the precise diagnosis of intracranial aneurysms (74), and with refinements in neurosurgical techniques surgical resection of ruptured and unruptured intracranial aneurysms may be carried out.

Necropsy investigations and clinical and angiographic studies have increased our understanding of the dynamics of the cerebral circulation. The extensive nature of the collateral circulation of the brain has now been outlined, as has the frequency with which extracerebral disease (stenosis or occlusion in the major arteries in the neck) may lead to extensive cerebrovascular dysfunction. Surgery is helpful in the treatment of selected cases, whereas altering the coagulability of the blood or platelet aggregation is useful in others.

Deficiency and Metabolic Disorders

The discovery of the therapeutic value of feeding liver to patients with pernicious anemia by Minot and Murphy in 1926 and the delineation of the role of the intrinsic gastric factor by Castle in 1928 brought about the first advances in the treatment of pernicious anemia (12,46). It was not until 1948, however, that cyanocobalamin or vitamin B_{12} was demonstrated to be many times more potent than concentrated liver in the treatment of the disease, and that its use could bring about complete hematologic and neurologic remission (61). The severe neurologic manifestations of pernicious anemia which were once seen with great frequency are now rarely encountered. Other deficiency diseases (e.g., scurvy, beriberi, and pellagra) have been fairly well understood for some time, although it was not until about 1935 that it was recognized that the polyneuritis associated with chronic alcoholism is actually the result of a thiamine deficiency and that it can be treated and reversed by the administration of that substance. It is also known now that other complications of chronic alcoholism (e.g., Korsakoff's and Wernicke's syndromes) are also secondary to thiamine deficiency and can be treated by thiamine administration (71).

Neuromuscular Disorders

Electromyography, which first assumed clinical importance around 1935, has gradually developed into an essential diagnostic technique. The more recently developed nerve conduction velocity studies have largely replaced testing for the reaction of degeneration, chronaxie determinations, and strength-duration curves, which were once used in the diagnosis of lower motor neuron, peripheral nerve, and neuromuscular disorders.

In an obituary note on the late Henry Viets, Robert Schwab stated that Viets, on his return to Boston from London in March 1935, had given

Schwab an ampule of a new drug, neostigmine, saying, "Find a myasthenia patient for tomorrow's conference and we will inject this into her muscles" (66). The effectiveness of the substance in bringing about relief of symptoms in myasthenia gravis had just been demonstrated by Mary Walker, and neostigmine was administered to a myasthenic patient in the United States for the first time on the next day, with results which greatly impressed and astounded the neurology staff present. Since that time it has become apparent that the disease may be diagnosed by a therapeutic test with either neostigmine (Prostigmin) or edrophonium (Tensilon), and major advances have been made in the treatment of the disorder.

Lumbosacral Pain

An outstanding contribution to neurologic diagnosis and treatment was the demonstration in 1934 by Mixter and Barr that a ruptured intervertebral disk is a common cause of low back pain with sciatic nerve or lumbosacral root radiation (48). At that time the neurologists, with their traditional views of sciatic neuralgia or neuritis, were slower than their surgical colleagues in appreciating the existence and importance of the ruptured intervertebral disk concept. Clifford Richardson, formerly chief neurologist at the University of Toronto, stated: "About 1937 Dr. Kenneth McKenzie [the neurosurgeon there] told me that these disc lesions were the most common cause of sciatica. I can well remember by disbelief and confident argument in favor of sciatic neuritis. Moreover, Dr. McKenzie had the temerity to challenge the existence of chronic brachial neuritis, suggesting that ruptured cervical intervertebral discs were the likely cause of the syndrome. Within a year or two I had climbed the disc bandwagon driven by the surgeons" (59). Doubtless this story, with different names for the principals, could be attributed to most other medical centers.

Headache and Head Pain

The important research by Harold Wolff and his associates as well as that of other investigators on the pathophysiology of headache and other head pain was carried out during the fourth and fifth decades of this century (77). This research made significant contributions to our understanding of mechanisms underlying many types of headache and have altered our understanding of the causes of head pain and our concepts of its therapy. Vascular headaches of the migraine type constitute a frequently encountered variety. In 1926 Maier demonstrated that ergotamine tartrate acted as a specific vasoconstrictor and was a potent therapeutic agent in many patients suffering from migraine headaches, acting to decrease the duration of the headache.

PSYCHIATRIC TREATMENT BY NEUROLOGISTS

With the development of electroconvulsive therapy for psychiatric ill-nesses, many neurologists who also treated mental patients adopted this method of treatment. With advances in psychopharmacology, however, and further observation of the side effects and complications of such therapy, its use was abandoned by neurologists. It is still carried out by some psy-chiatrists, however, but infrequently.

The observation that lesions of the frontal lobes may decrease emotional and affective responses and relieve anxiety and nervous tension led to the development of the operation of prefrontal leukotomy or lobotomy for the treatment of emotional disorders (29). Various modifications of this proce-dure were developed to section the association fibers from the prefrontal region to the subcortical gray masses, especially the thalamus and hypothalamus. This was done in large numbers of patients with manic-depressive psychosis, schizophrenia, and obsessive-compulsive states; it was also used to decrease the reaction to intractable pain of organic origin, and later to treat uncontrollable violence and rage. An immense literature on the subject accumulated during the late 1930s and the 1940s. A technique that could be done as an office procedure, transorbital lobotomy, was even used. Physicians soon became disillusioned by the untoward consequences of such psychosurgery, however, and the technique lost favor almost as rapidly as it had gained it. This was an unhappy chapter in the history of the neurologic sciences.

NEUROLOGISTS AND NEUROSCIENTISTS OF THE PERIOD

Neurology and the neurologic sciences developed so rapidly in the United States during the second quarter of the twentieth century, and so many individuals played significant roles in their development, that it is not feasi-ble in this small volume to include detailed biographic sketches of all of them. However, those whose contributions were most significant are dis-cussed briefly.

Neuroanatomists and Neurophysiologists

Gotthelf Carl Huber (1865–1934) was born in India, the son of Swiss missionaries (38). When he was 6 years old the family moved to the United States, where his father held pastorates in several midwestern churches. He entered the University of Michigan Medical School, from which he graduated in 1887. Following graduation he was appointed assistant dem-onstrator in anatomy at the University of Michigan and continued serving Michigan for 47 years. He did, however, spend 1 year studying in Berlin, 1 year in Prague, and 1 year (1911–1912) serving as professor of embryology at the Wistar Institute of Anatomy and Biology. He was active in research and teaching in embryology, histology, and neuroanatomy. For many years he was professor of anatomy and director of the anatomic laboratories at Michigan, and at the time of his death he was also Dean of the School of Graduate Studies. He never allowed his many administrative responsibilities, however, to interfere with his teaching activities or investigative work. In 1920 he became associated with C. U. Ariëns Kappers, Director of the Central Institute for Brain Research in Amsterdam, and assisted him in the completion of his *Vergleichende Anatomie des Nerven Systems der Wirbeltiere und des Menschen;* this was later translated into English and published in 1935 under the title *The Comparative Anatomy of the Nervous System of Vertebrates Including Man,* with Ariëns Kappers, Huber, and Crosby as co-authors (2).

Huber had been joined in 1920 by Elizabeth C. Crosby, who was born in Petersburg, Michigan, in 1888, was graduated from Adrian College, and received her Ph.D. degree in neuroanatomy from the University of Chicago under C. Judson Herrick in 1915. She was an active collaborator of Huber as well as an original investigator on her own. After the death of Huber in 1934, she completed the text of their book, read and edited the proof, and is responsible for the finished two-volume book. She continues with her investigations and writing, and the textbook written by her and her associates, *Correlative Anatomy of the Nervous System* (17), is widely used.

Rex Branville Harrison (1870–1959) was an experimental embryologist and a neuroembryologist (62). For many years he was chairman of the undergraduate and graduate zoology departments at Yale University and after his retirement was chairman of the National Research Council (1938–1946). His early transplantation studies on tadpole nerves convinced him that nerve fibers are outgrowths of single neurons. In 1907 he reported the first successful animal tissue culture.

George Coghill (1872–1941) was professor of anatomy at the University of Kansas from 1913 to 1925, and during the next 10 years was research professor of comparative anatomy at the Wistar Institute of Anatomy and Biology (41). He intensively studied the relationship between embryologic development and behavior, choosing the salamander as his research subject and recording the exact sequence of changes in its behavior from first motility to the adult stage. He was a member of the editorial board of the *Journal of Comparative Neurology* from 1904 until his death, and was managing editor from 1927 until 1933.

Joseph Erlanger (1874–1965) was graduated from the Johns Hopkins Medical School, following which he served an internship in medicine under William Osler, a fellowship in pathology under William H. Welch, and an assistantship in physiology under William H. Howell (3). Langley and Anderson had stated in 1904 that the central end of an efferent somatic nerve fiber can make functional union with the peripheral end of any preganglionic nerve, and in 1905 Erlanger provided evidence for this by suturing a spinal nerve to the peripheral end of the cut vagus nerve; stimulation of the nerve produced inhibition of the heart. In 1910 he was appointed professor of physiology at Washington University in St. Louis. There, working with Herbert Gasser, he studied the highly differentiated function of single nerve fibers and developed the present standard classification of nerve fibers. Erlanger and Gasser were awarded the Nobel Prize in Physiology in 1944 for this work.

Stephen Walter Ransom (1880–1942) developed his interest in neurology during his student years by his association with J. B. Johnston at the University of Minnesota and H. H. Donaldson at the University of Chicago (43). He began a long-term study for his doctoral thesis which revealed the presence of nonmyelinated fibers in peripheral nerves. He clarified the hypothalamic innervation of the pituitary gland and established its importance in water exchange and gonadotropic control. Over a period of many years he made significant contributions to our understanding of the anatomy and functions of the hypothalamus. He was professor of anatomy at Northwestern University for many years, and later was director of an Institute of Neurology there. His textbook *The Anatomy of the Nervous System,* which first appeared in 1920, has been republished in many revisions and editions (57).

James W. Papez (1883–1958) was professor of anatomy at Cornell University in Ithaca, New York, from 1920 to 1951 (36). He expressed the belief that emotions are phylogenetically related to gustation and olfaction, and he conceived a "mechanism for emotion," the hippocampo-mammillo-thalamo-cingulate-hippocampal circuit (52). He established the concept of the limbic lobe—the hippocampal gyrus, uncus, isthmus, gyrus cinguli, and related areas. He observed that these structures, through their connections with the hypothalamus and thalamus, play an important part in the central regulation of the autonomic nervous system and of visceral and sexual functions, as well as in the autonomic factors involved in emotional expression, but his observations long went unrecognized.

Andrew T. Rasmussen (1883–1954) was born in Utah and was graduated from Brigham Young University where he taught biology from 1909 to 1913 (10). He then entered graduate study at Cornell University, where he received his Ph.D. degree in 1916. He entered the anatomy department at the University of Minnesota, and in 1925 succeeded J. B. Johnston as professor of neuroanatomy, a post he held until 1952. His major contributions dealt with the anatomy of the hypophysis. He was an excellent artist, and his lucid and instructive diagrams add to his books *Outlines of Neuroanatomy* and *The Principal Nervous Pathways* (58).

Johannes Gregorius Dusser de Barenne (1885–1940) was born in The Netherlands and received his medical degree from Amsterdam University (30). His professional career then began in the physiology laboratory of that university where he studied the effect of strychnine on the reflex activity of invertebrate ganglia. He then began a study of decerebrate rigidity, tonic neck and vestibular reflexes, and posture. From 1918 to 1930 he was associated with Rudolf Magnus in this study at Utrecht University. Disturbed by the religious restrictions of the Dutch universities, he moved to the United States, and from 1930 until his premature death in 1940 he was on the faculty of the Yale School of Medicine, where he engaged in active research. His primary contribution during this period lay in the introduction of the new technique of physiologic neuronography, which has made possible a vast research endeavor involving analysis of the interaction of various cortical and subcortical areas of the brain.

Olof Larsell (1886–1964) was born in Sweden and emigrated to the Pacific Northwest as a small boy (20). He was graduated from Linfield College, where he taught biology for 5 years. He carried out graduate study at Northwestern University and then under C. Judson Herrick at the University of Chicago, where he received his Ph.D. degree in 1918. Herrick stimulated his interest in comparative neuroanatomy. His major field of investigation was the cerebellum, and he made many significant contributions to our understanding of its structure and functions (40). He taught neuroanatomy at the University of Oregon from 1921 to 1952 and was working on a monumental monograph, *The Cerebellum from Myxinoids to Man,* at the time of his death.

Herbert Spencer Gasser (1888–1963), while still a medical student, was inspired by the lectures of Joseph Erlanger (37). After his graduation from medical school he served for 1 year as an instructor in physiology at the University of Wisconsin after which he was invited by Erlanger, then at Washington University, to join him. The two remained closely associated from 1916 to 1932. Together they developed the cathode ray oscilloscope, by means of which they could study the action potentials of nerve fibers. They were jointly awarded the Nobel Prize in Physiology in 1944 for their study of the anatomy and physiology of individual nerve fibers. In 1932 Gasser went to the New York Hospital-Cornell Medical Center as professor of physiology, and 3 years later he was called to the Rockefeller Institute to succeed Simon Flexner as director.

Sam Lillard Clark (1896–1920) was born in Nashville, Tennessee. After graduating from Vanderbilt University, he entered the laboratory of Stephen Ransom at Northwestern University, where he worked in neuroanatomy and neurophysiology (68). He then went to Washington University in St. Louis and obtained a Ph.D. degree, after which he returned to Vanderbilt University to teach neuroanatomy and engage in research. Clark made important contributions to our understanding of the neurophysiology of the cerebellum and the mechanisms of cerebral concussion. He edited the later editions of Ransom's textbook after that author's death. He was president of the

American Association of Anatomy during 1950 to 1952 and was editor of the *American Journal of Anatomy* at the time of his death.

John Farquhar Fulton (1899–1960) was born in Minnesota and was graduated from Yale University, following which he went to Oxford University as a Rhodes Scholar (9). He remained at Oxford for 4 years and received the degrees of B.A., M.A., and Ph.D. there. Oxford later awarded him the honorary degree of Doctor of Science in 1941 and that of Doctor of Literature in 1957. At Oxford he studied under Charles Sherrington, who helped to develop his interest in neurophysiology. Returning to the United States, he received the degree of Doctor of Medicine from Harvard University in 1927, following which he served as an assistant in neurosurgery under Harvey Cushing at the Peter Bent Brigham Hospital. In 1929 he was appointed Sterling Professor of Physiology at Yale University, a post he actually assumed in 1931. Because of ill health, he retired from the chair of physiology in 1951 and was appointed Sterling Professor of the History of Medicine, a post he held until his death. He made so many contributions to neurophysiology it is difficult to state which were the most important. Paul Bucy has said that the most important one was his role in the development of prefrontal lobotomy. After he and his pupil Carlyle Jacobsen demonstrated the effect of the procedure on a "neurotic" chimpanzee at an international meeting in London, Egas Moniz returned to Lisbon and performed it for the treatment of behavioral disturbances in humans (29). This form of treatment is no longer in vogue, but research relative to it added significantly to our knowledge of cerebral function. Others believe that his most important contribution was his training program in neurophysiology at Yale University, his *Physiology of the Nervous System* (27), or his work on muscle tone and contraction. He also wrote extensively on medical history and in 1946 published a biography of Harvey Cushing (28).

Neurologists

Israel Strauss (1873–1955) received his medical degree from the College of Physicians and Surgeons (75). After an internship in the Mount Sinai Hospital he spent 2 years in Vienna studying histology and pathology. On his return to New York he joined the staff of the Mount Sinai Hospital, first on the medical service and then as a neurologist. In 1925 he became chief of the neurology service, a position he held until his retirement in 1938. In 1920 he organized a neuropathology laboratory at Mount Sinai Hospital, which was subsequently under the direction of J. H. Globus. He published papers on the treatment of syphilis, the etiology and pathology of acute poliomyelitis, and the etiology of encephalitis lethargica.

Harold Douglas Singer (1875–1940) was born in London, England, and received his medical education at St. Thomas's Hospital and the University of London (33). After a residency at the National Hospital, Queen Square, he returned to St. Thomas's Hospital as resident physician. He came to the United States in 1904 and was first associate professor of neurology at Creighton University Medical School in Omaha, Nebraska, and then associate professor of psychiatry at the University of Nebraska. He was director of the Illinois State Psychiatric Institute from 1907 to 1920, and in 1921 was appointed professor and chief of the department of psychiatry at the College of Medicine of the University of Illinois. He was editor-in-chief of the *Archives of Neurology and Psychiatry* from 1934 until his death in 1940, and was the first president of the American Board of Psychiatry, serving from its establishment in 1934 until the time of his death.

William Biddle Cadwalader (1876–1957) was graduated from Princeton University and received a medical degree from the University of Pennsylvania (44). Following 3 years at the Pennsylvania Hospital he did postgraduate work in Vienna and Munich. During his early years he published a number of papers, including pathologic studies on acute poliomyelitis, experimental work on the anterolateral column of the spinal cord, and studies on cerebral hemorrhage and infarction. He served from 1917 to 1919 with the American Expeditionary Forces as a neurologist in base hospitals in France, and rose from the rank of captain to that of lieutenant colonel. His experiences in the war led him to write the chapter "The Pathology of Gunshot Wounds and Other Severe Injuries of the Nervous System" in Keen's *Surgery* in 1921. In 1920 he became an associate in neurology at the University of Pennsylvania, where he was promoted to the rank of clinical professor in 1932. His major contribution to neurology was his 1932 book *Diseases of the Spinal Cord.*

Walter Frank Schaller (1879–1970) was graduated from the Cooper Union Medical College, San Francisco (later the Stanford University Medical School) in 1902 (24). Following a few years in the United States Navy, he spent 3 years doing postgraduate work in Europe. During this time he became interested in diseases of the nervous system and studied under Widal, Dejerine, and Babinski. Returning to San Francisco he became one of the pioneer neurologists on the West Coast. From 1911 until his retirement in 1945 he was on the faculty of the Stanford University Medical School as professor of medicine, division of neuropsychiatry. His publications dealt mainly with clinical presentations, some with associated pathologic confirmation.

James Bourne Ayer (1882–1963) was graduated from Harvard Medical School in 1907, following which he began his clinical work at the Massachusetts General Hospital (19). He had an early interest in cytologic studies of the CSF. During World War I he served in the United States Army Medical Corps and was assigned to a special group based at The Johns Hopkins Hospital. This group, under the direction of Lewis Weed, was asked to study the severe outbreaks of meningococcal meningitis in training camps. The use of puncture of the cisterna magna to obtain CSF in experimental animals encouraged Ayer and his associates to develop a safe technique for doing so in humans, which was first reported in 1917 (73). On his return to the Massachusetts General Hospital in 1919, he elaborated the technique, and by 1921 had, by careful measurements at combined lumbar and cisterna punctures, established the criteria of spinal block of the subarachnoid space. Ayer had first received an appointment at the Harvard Medical School in 1910 and an outpatient staff appointment at the Massachusetts General Hospital in 1911. After World War I Ayer set up a special cerebrospinal fluid (CSF) laboratory at the hospital where normal standards were established and the Denis-Ayer method of quantitative estimation of the protein content of the CSF was introduced. By 1923 he could report on nearly 2,000 cisterna punctures. In 1925 he defined criteria for pressure measurements for the recognition of lateral sinus thrombosis (the Ayer-Tobey test). In 1926 E. Wyllys Taylor retired and Ayer succeeded him as James Jackson Putnam Professor of Neurology at Harvard Medical School, a post he held until his retirement.

William Gordon Lennox (1884 – 1960) was born in Colorado and received his medical degree from Harvard Medical School in 1913 (13). After 3 years of hospital work, mostly at the Massachusetts General Hospital, he went to Peking, China, where he spent 1 year learning the language and then 3 years at the newly organized Rockefeller Medical School and Hospital. In 1922 he returned to Boston and received an appointment in the department of neuropathology of Harvard Medical School and began the project that he was to be engaged in for the rest of his life—a pursuit of the causes and treatment of epilepsy. In the beginning he worked with Stanley Cobb on research supported by the Rockefeller Foundation. Later with Cobb and Harold Wolff he studied cerebral blood flow and the effect on pial vessels of variations in the oxygen and carbon dioxide content of the blood. Around 1934, with Hallowell Davis and Frederic and Erna Gibbs, he studied the newly developed electroencephalographic techniques in neurologic diseases and especially in epilepsy. He wrote many papers and several books describing his research on epilepsy. His major work, the two-volume *Epilepsy and Related Disorders,* which he wrote with his daughter Margaret Lennox-Buchtal, was published just a few weeks before his death. He received many honors, and his work was well received by his contemporaries. The Gibbses dedicated their *Atlas of Electroencephalography* to him, stating: "He is the good physician in modern dress, the humanitarian scientist, whose resolute high purpose, wisdom, gentleness, and simplicity have beaten the devil out of epilepsy."

Israel Spanier Wechsler (1886 – 1962) was born in Romania but came to the United States as a boy (76). He received his medical degree from New York University in 1907. After some time in general practice, he trained at the Neurological Institute under Frederick Tilney. He became chief of neurology at the Vanderbilt Clinic in 1919 and professor of clinical neurology at the College of Physicians and Surgeons in 1931. He was attending neurologist at the Montefiore Hospital from 1920 to 1938 and chief of the neurology service at the Mount Sinai Hospital from 1938 to 1951. His *Text Book of Clinical Neurology,* first published in 1927, was widely read and went through nine editions. Wechsler added a chapter on the history of neurology to the last edition. He read and spoke several languages, and wrote extensively on the history of medicine.

Lewis John Pollock (1886–1966) was born in Russia and came to the United States as a boy (18). He received his medical degree from the University of Illinois in 1906 and became associated with Hugh T. Patrick in the practice of neurology in Chicago and in teaching neurology at the Northwestern University Medical School. During World War I he was neurologist at one base hospital in France and neurologic consultant at another. He was known for his skills as a neurologist, research-oriented clinician, and teacher. His contributions to the diagnosis and symptomatology of peripheral nerve lesions complement the classic descriptions of Weir Mitchell; his clinical and physiologic studies of human spinal cord injuries were major contributions, and his analyses of the reflex influences on decerebrate rigidity were based on sound anatomic facts.

Henry Alsop Riley (1887–1966) (Fig. 26) was graduated from Yale University and the College of Physicians and Surgeons (45). His entire professional life was associated with the College of Physicians and Surgeons of Columbia University. He was appointed instructor in neurology in 1916, advancing to the position of professor of clinical neurology in 1939, a position he held until appointed professor emeritus on his retirement in 1953. After the affiliation of the Neurological Institute with the Columbia-Presbyterian Medical Center, his teaching and investigative activities were confined to the wards of the Neurological Institute and the laboratories in the adjacent College of Physicians and Surgeons. His interest in the anatomy and physiology of the nervous system was kindled by Frederick Tilney, with whom he wrote his major contribution *The Form and Functions of the Central Nervous System: An Introduction to the Study of Nervous Diseases* (1920). He also wrote *An Atlas of the Basal Ganglia, Brain Stem and Spinal Cord Based on Myelin Stained Material* (1943) and contributed chapters to Tilney's book *The Brain from Ape to Man* (1928). He was secretary of the American Neurological Association from 1922 to 1946 and president in 1947, as well as secretary-general of the First International Neurological Congress (held in Berne, Switzerland, in 1931) and either vice-president or honorary president of all of the following congresses until 1965.

Stanley Cobb (1887–1968) (Fig. 27) attended Harvard College and Harvard Medical School, from which he graduated in 1914 (1). After a surgical internship under Cushing at the Peter Bent Brigham Hospital, he did postgraduate work in physiology and psychiatry at Johns Hopkins University.

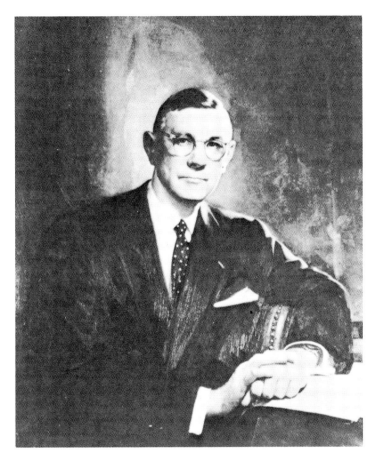

FIG. 26. Henry A. Riley. (From ref. 45.)

During World War I he served in the United States Army Medical Corps, after which he returned to Boston and was appointed instructor in physiology and neurology at Harvard Medical School and assistant neurologist at the Massachusetts General Hospital. He was appointed assistant professor of neuropathology in 1920 and associate professor in 1923. Having been chosen to establish a course in neuropathology, he was sent to Europe by the Rockefeller Foundation and studied in Oxford, London, Paris, and Berlin. Upon his return to Boston he was appointed chief of the neurology service at the Boston City Hospital, with a substantial grant from the Rockefeller Foundation, and a year later was appointed Bullard Professor of Neuropathology at the Harvard Medical School. While at the Boston City Hospitals, Cobb was associated with William Lennox, Frank Fremont-Smith, Tracy Putnam, H. Houston Merritt, Frederick Gibbs, and others, all

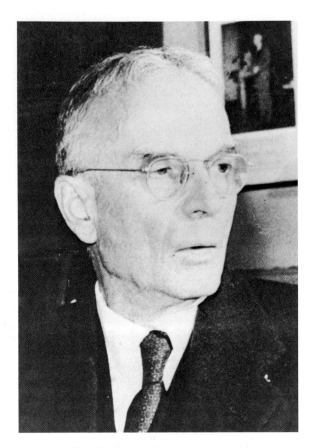

FIG. 27. Stanley Cobb. (From ref. 1.)

of whom made significant contributions to the neurologic sciences. In 1934 he transferred to the Massachusetts General Hospital, where he was the first chief of psychiatry; he also continued as Bullard Professor of Neuropathology, holding both posts until his retirement in 1954. He was a gifted writer and wrote on a wide range of neurologic and psychiatric subjects.

Henry William Woltman (1889–1964) received his medical degree from the University of Minnesota in 1913 and received the degree of Ph.D. in neurology from the same university 4 years later (51). His interest in neurology was influenced by Arthur S. Hamilton, professor of neurology. He was appointed assistant in neurology at the Mayo Clinic in Rochester, Minnesota, in 1917, and the next year was promoted to the rank of instructor. Through successive promotions he achieved the rank of professor of neurology at the Mayo Clinic and the Graduate School of Medicine of the University of Minnesota in 1931. In 1930 he succeeded Walter D. Shelden as chairman of the section of neurology and psychiatry at the Clinic. At many medical centers during the 1930s clinical neurology was either disappearing into the pathology laboratories or being absorbed into the fields of psychiatry or neurosurgery. Under Woltman's leadership, however, neurology remained a separate entity at the Mayo Clinic and provided an essential role in patient care, residency training, and clinical research. In 1946 he initiated and supported the development of a separate section of psychiatry at the Clinic. His doctoral thesis dealt with the brain changes in pernicious anemia. He made significant contributions to the pathology of diabetic neuropathy and wrote extensively on the peripheral neuropathies, especially those associated with systemic diseases, as well as on diseases of the spinal cord.

Johannes Maagaard Nielsen (1890–1969) was born in Denmark, and came to the United States at the age of five (72). After working as a carpenter and construction foreman, he became disenchanted with his work and decided on a medical career. After premedical studies in night school he entered the University of Chicago Medical School, from which he was graduated with honors in 1923. He interned at the Los Angeles County General Hospital where he became acquainted with Samuel D. Ingham, who encouraged his interest in neurology. His postgraduate training was done in Vienna, and in 1929 he entered the practice of neurology and psychiatry with Ingham. He accepted an appointment on the Neurology Service of the Los Angeles County General Hospital and lectured in neurology at the College of Medical Evangelists (now Loma Linda University). When the University of Southern California Medical School was reopened in 1931, he was appointed associate professor of neurology and psychiatry. He succeeded Ingham as professor and head of the department in 1945, resigning in 1952 because he opposed the pending separation of psychiatry from neurology. His influence on the development of neurology in southern California was prodigious. He was instrumental, along with Ingham, Carl W. Rand, and Cyril B. Courville, in developing the Los Angeles Neurological Society and in publishing its *Bulletin.* He was an incessant and productive worker, using as his base the large amount of clinical and pathologic material available to him at the Los Angeles County General Hospital. With Courville he wrote a series of comprehensive reports of the intracranial complications of otogenous infections. His interest in cerebral localization led to publication of his monograph *Agnosia, Apraxia and Aphasia: Their Value in Cerebral Localization* (1936). He was author of *A Textbook of Neurology,* published in 1941 and revised in 1946 and 1951. He contributed chapters to a number of reference books and textbooks.

Henry R. Viets (1890–1969) was born in Massachusetts and graduated from Dartmouth College and Harvard Medical School (66). Because of his interest in the history of medicine he was awarded a Mosely Traveling Fellowship, and he went to Oxford for a year where he worked with Osler and

Sherrington. He spent 2 years in the Medical Corps of the United States Army, rising to the rank of major. In 1919 he was appointed to the neurology department of Harvard Medical School and the Massachusetts General Hospital, and remained in these positions until he was awarded emeritus status in 1941. His major clinical interest was myasthenia gravis, and he established the myasthenia gravis clinic at the Massachusetts General Hospital. It was under him that neostigmine was first used to diagnose and treat myasthenia gravis in the United States (66). When the Myasthenia Gravis Foundation was established in 1962 he was made chairman of its medical advisory board; the Foundation annually awards student fellowships named after him. He continued his interest and writing on the history of medicine, was active in the Boston Medical Library, and served on the editorial board of the *New England Journal of Medicine* from 1927 to 1966.

Hans Heinrich Reese (1891–1973) was born in Germany and received his undergraduate and medical education there (26). He was awarded a medical degree from the University of Kiel in 1917, following which he studied pathology, internal medicine, and neurology at the University of Hamburg. Interested in the treatment of neurosyphilis, he came to the United States where he became acquainted with Hideyo Noguchi and Bernard Sachs. Through them he met William Lorenz, chairman of the department of neuropsychiatry at the University of Wisconsin, who offered him a position as assistant professor in 1924. He became a full professor in 1929 and was chairman of the department in 1940 and again from 1954 to 1956. When psychiatry and neurology were separated in 1956, he remained with neurology and was chairman of the department of neurology until his retirement in 1958. He made many contributions to American and international neurology.

Percival Bailey (1892–1973), who had to work to pay his way through college and medical school, in 1918 was awarded a Ph.D. degree from the University of Chicago and an M.D. degree from Northwestern University (8). After an internship in Mercy Hospital in Chicago he spent several years in neurosurgery with Harvey Cushing at the Peter Bent Brigham Hospital in Boston. Following this he studied neuropathology under George Hassin, neurology under Pierre Marie, psychiatry under Pierre Janet, and neurophysiology under Frederic Bremer and Georges Schaltenbrand. In 1928 he went to the University of Chicago, where he created the division of neurology and neurologic surgery. Frustrated by administrative restrictions, he left 11 years later and went to the University of Illinois where he was professor of neurology and neurologic surgery. Following studies on psychomotor epilepsy with Frederick A. Gibbs, his interests turned again to psychiatry, and he accepted appointments as director of the Illinois State Psychopathic Institute and professor of psychiatry at the University of Illinois. He induced Illinois to build the Illinois State Psychiatric Institute and to establish an authority for psychiatric training and research. He published extensively on neurology, neurosurgery, neuropathology, and psychiatry.

Harold George Wolff (1898–1962) attended Harvard College and Harvard Medical School where he came under the influence of Stanley Cobb, who provided him with a sound knowledge of the nervous system (35). After clinical work at the Roosevelt Hospital and Cornell Clinic in New York City, he returned to Harvard to pursue research on the cerebral circulation under the guidance of Henry S. Forbes. Here he worked with Lennox, Cobb, and others. His attempts to understand the relationship of the network of nerves surrounding the cerebral blood vessels led to his exhaustive study of headache and head pain (77). At the Phipps Psychiatric Clinic in Baltimore he collaborated with Horsley Gantt in a study of the conditioned reflex. His work with Adolf Meyer, also at Phipps, contributed to the development of his unified concept of the mind-body relationship. He worked for a year in Graz, Austria, with Otto Loewi on neurohumeral transmission and did further work on the conditioned reflex with Ivan Pavlov in Leningrad. When New York Hospital-Cornell Medical Center was opened, Wolff was placed in charge of neurology, and later, when Foster Kennedy retired, he also took charge of the neurology service at Bellevue Hospital. A grateful patient of his endowed a chair at Cornell Medical School, and he was named the Anne Parrish Titzell Professor of Medicine in Neurology. He published 539 papers and 14 books and monographs, written either alone or with collaborators. He was appointed editor-in-chief of the *Archives of Neurology and Psychiatry* in 1956 and continued in this position when the journal became the *Archives of Neurology* in 1959. His honors were many.

Roland Parks Mackay (1900–1968) (Fig. 28) was born in Georgia but spent his early years in Canada (7). He received his medical degree from the University of Toronto in 1925, his training in neurology at the Mayo Clinic, and his training in neuropathology in Germany. He practiced neurology in Chicago from 1929 until the time of his death. He also served on the faculty of Rush Medical College (1929–1933), the University of Illinois College of Medicine (1934–1961), and Northwestern University Medical School (1961–1968). He was editor of the section on neurology in the *Year Book of Neurology, Psychiatry and Neurosurgery* from 1949 to 1968 and served on the editorial board of the *Archives of Neurology* and *Neurology*. He was active in neurologic affairs, and his contributions to neurology were many.

Derek Ernest Denny-Brown (1901–1981) was born in Christchurch, New Zealand (25) and received his medical education at Otago University. Interested in problems of posture and movement, he served as Beit Fellow in Sherrington's laboratory at Oxford from 1925 to 1928. Turning to clinical neurology, he served as resident medical officer at the National Hospital, Queen Square, London, from 1928 to 1931 and then as registrar at Guy's Hospital from 1931 to 1935. There he was under the guidance of Charles Symonds but spent one half of each day in neuropathology with Godwin Greenfield. He continued his neurophysiologic studies both in animals and humans. He spent some time in John Fulton's laboratory at Yale University

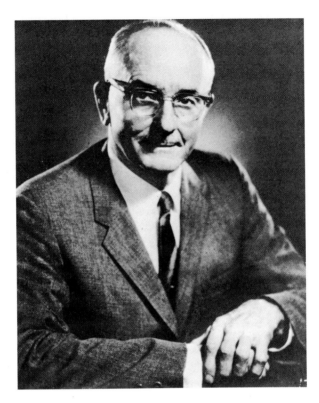

FIG. 28. Roland P. Mackay. (From ref. 7.)

studying the frontal lobes in monkeys. In 1935 he was appointed assistant physician at the National Hospital, and the same year he was appointed neurologist at St. Bartholomew's Hospital. In 1939 he was offered and accepted the post of chief of the neurology service at the Boston City Hospital. He still held a commission in the British Army, however, and when Great Britain was drawn into World War II, he was called to organize the medical service of a military hospital for head injuries. In 1941 this task was completed, and, at the request of Harvard Medical School and the Office of Scientific Research and Development, he was released to serve on the Committee on Aviation Medicine of the Office of Scientific Research and Development in Washington. This was a part-time position and he was also able to accept the positions of professor of neurology at Harvard Medical School and director of the neurology unit at the Boston City Hospital. In 1944 he was recalled to active duty, and served in India. In May 1946 he returned to Harvard and Boston and was named the James Jackson Putnam Professor of Neurology, a position he held until his retirement in 1967, at which time he was made chief of the section on neurophysiology and associate director of the New England Regional Primate Research Center. In 1977 he became a Fogarty Scholar-in-Residence at the National Institutes of Health in Bethesda, Maryland, where he had the opportunity to write up the reports of the last 5 years of his research in neurophysiology. His research covered a wide range of clinical disorders and neurophysiologic problems, including a systematic investigation of disorders of posture and movement, and experiments on the nature of reflex activity, spasticity, involuntary movements, and dystonia. Among his major publications are *Selected Writings of Sir Charles Sherrington* (1939), *The Frontal Lobes and Their Function* (1941), *The Basal Ganglia and Their Relation to Disorders of Movement* (1962), and *The Cerebral Control of Movement* (1966). *Diseases of Muscle: A Study in Pathology* (1962) was written with R. D. Adams and C. M. Pearson. He was the senior editor of the *Centennial Anniversary Volume of the American Neurological Association 1875–1975.*

Richard Biddle Richter (1901–1971) was born in La Porte, Indiana, and educated at the University of Chicago and Rush College of Medicine (67). After an internship in the Presbyterian Hospital in Chicago, he became a junior faculty member at Rush, acting as assistant to Thor Rothstein and Peter Bassoe. (Rothstein had been a pupil of Gustaf Retzius in Stockholm, and Bassoe had trained in neurology under Hugh Patrick.) In 1936 Richter was invited to join the recently established full-time faculty at the University of Chicago. He accepted the invitation and remained there as chief of the division of neurology until his retirement 30 years later. His contributions to neurology were numerous, appearing mainly in the form of neuropathologic reports based on studies that were meticulously carried out and clearly presented in Richter's exceptional literary style.

Hiram Houston Merritt (1902–1978) (Fig. 29) was born in North Carolina and attended public schools there and the University of North Carolina (11). He completed his undergraduate education at Vanderbilt University and in 1926 received his medical degree from The Johns Hopkins University. He trained in medicine at the New Haven Hospital and in neurology and neuropathology at the Boston City Hospital and in Munich. During his 13 years in Boston he rose to the rank of associate professor of neurology in Harvard Medical School. It was at the Boston City Hospital that he and Tracy Putnam did their experimental studies on anticonvulsant drugs that led to the discovery of diphenylhydantoin sodium (phenytoin), which revolutionized the treatment of epilepsy. It was there also that he and Frank Fremont-Smith did their detailed study of the CSF which led to the publication of their book in 1937. At Boston City Hospital and at the Boston Psychopathic Hospital, he, Raymond D. Adams, and Harry C. Solomon did their work of neurosyphilis, leading to the publication of their book on the subject in 1946.

In 1944 Merritt moved to New York City and began his long association with Columbia University. The first 4 years were spent at the Montefiore

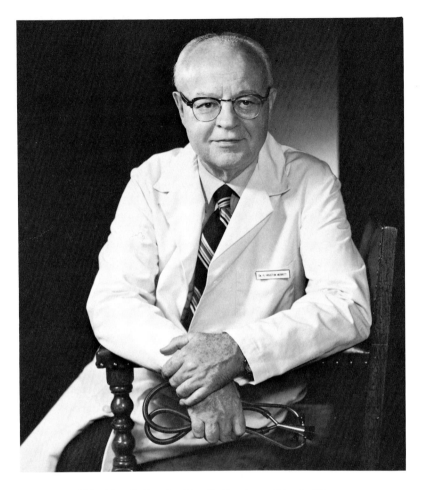

FIG. 29.   H. Houston Merritt. *Courtesy of* Karsh, Ottawa.

Hospital where he was chief of the division of neuropsychiatry. In 1948 he was appointed professor and chairman of the department of neurology at the College of Physicians and Surgeons and director of the neurology service at the Neurological Institute, Columbia-Presbyterian Medical Center. He held these two posts for 23 years, a period in which there was tremendous growth of neurology as a specialty at Columbia and in the United States. In 1958 he was appointed acting dean of the College of Physicians and Surgeons and acting vice president for medical affairs of Columbia University, receiving permanent appointments the following year. He held these offices until his retirement at the age of 68 in 1970. He continued to be active in clinical affairs, teaching, and research in spite of his administrative duties. His *A Textbook of Neurology*, first published in 1955, was printed in five editions.

Despite his commitments to the medical school and hospital, Merritt found time to serve the United States government in a number of important advisory posts and to participate in the activities of many voluntary health agencies. He was an initial and long-time member of the National Advisory Council of the National Institute of Neurological Diseases and Blindness, now the National Institute of Neurological and Communicative Disorders and Stroke; he served as a consultant to the U.S. Army, Navy, and Veterans Administration; and he was active on the advisory boards of the National Multiple Sclerosis Society, the United Cerebral Palsy Association, the Muscular Dystrophy Association of America, the Myasthenia Gravis Foundation, and the Epilepsy Foundation of America. He was an outstanding leader among the group of people who contributed to the dramatic growth of neurology in the United States during the past half-century.

Samuel Bernard Wortis (1904–1969) was born in Brooklyn and educated at New York University and Cornell University Medical College, from which he was graduated in 1927 (46). He was a believer that neurology and psychiatry should be firmly based on internal medicine, and was a diplomate of the American Board of Internal Medicine as well as of the American Board of Psychiatry and Neurology, where he was certified in neurology and psychiatry. He taught briefly at Johns Hopkins, Columbia, and Cornell Universities, but most of his professional career was spent with New York University and Bellevue Hospital. His first appointment in 1931 was as director of laboratory and experimental neuropsychiatry. In 1942 he was appointed professor and chairman of the department of neuropsychiatry. From 1960 to 1963 he was also dean of the medical school. He was coeditor of the *Year Book of Neurology, Neurosurgery and Psychiatry* from 1954 to 1969, when he became the first editor of the *Year Book of Psychiatry*. His research interests were diverse, ranging from metabolic studies on excised brain tissue to problems of alcoholism and drug addiction.

James Lee O'Leary (1904–1975), born in Wisconsin, received degrees of bachelor of science (1925), doctor of philosophy (1928), and doctor of medicine (1931) from the University of Chicago (42). There he came under the influence of G. W. Bartelmez, R. R. Bensley, and C. Judson Herrick, who stimulated his interest in the nervous system and in research. While an instructor in anatomy at the University of Chicago he was offered a position as assistant professor of anatomy (neuroanatomy) at Washington University in St. Louis, where he began a collaboration with George Bishop and Peter Heinbecker that was to continue for many years. He began his research on the histologic and functional studies of somatic and autonomic nerves and later, with Bishop, turned his interest to the cerebral cortex. For almost 30 years O'Leary personally trained almost every resident in neurosurgery and neurology at Washington University in the techniques of research and electroencephalography. In 1943 he entered the Armed Services and at the Mason General Hospital in Brentwood, New York, taught neuroanatomy, neurophysiology, and electroencephalography. Following discharge from the military, he returned to Washington University School of Medicine where he was made professor and chairman of the department of neurology and chief of neurology at Barnes Hospital.

Neuropathologists

Cobb, Bailey, Alpers, Richter, and others were also neuropathologists and wrote extensively on the subject. Among those who more or less limited their work to neuropathology are the following:

George B. Hassin (1873–1951), born in Russia, received his medical training there and then spent 4 years studying and working with general pathology (34). Becoming interested in neuropathology, he went to Vienna in 1901 to work under Obersteiner and Marburg. Here he met a number of young American neurologists who encouraged him to emigrate to the United States. He moved to Chicago where he at first entered general practice but then turned to neurology; through the influence of Patrick and Bassoe he received an appointment as attending neurologist at Cook County Hospital. A year later he spent some time with Alfons Jakob in Hamburg but then returned to Chicago, limiting his work to clinical neurology and neuropathology. Appointed professor of clinical neurology at the University of Illinois Medical College, his contributions covered almost every phase of neuropathology. In 1933 he published the first edition of his textbook on neuropathology, which had two subsequent editions. He, with Joseph H. Globus, Armando Ferraro, and Arthur Weil, was instrumental in establishing the *Journal of Neuropathology and Experimental Neurology*, and was its first editor, serving for 9 years.

Joseph H. Globus (1885–1952) was born in Russia but educated in the United States (23), where he graduated from Columbia University and Cornell University Medical School. For more than 30 years he was consulting neurologist at Mount Sinai Hospital in New York City and director of the neuropathology laboratory there. His major contribution to neuropathology dealt with the classification of brain tumors and a study of vascular diseases of the nervous system. He succeeded Hassin as editor of the *Journal of Neuropathology and Experimental Neurology* and also served for many years as editor of the *Journal of the Mount Sinai Hospital*.

Arthur Weil (1887–1969) was born in Germany, where he began his medical and scientific career (60). His early interests were physiological chemistry and endocrinology. In 1922 he emigrated to New York City and joined the pathology department of Montefiore Hospital where he served for 3 years as resident in neuropathology. He continued to work in neuropathology and also in neuroanatomy. In 1928 Stephen W. Ransom asked him to join the staff of the Neurological Institute of Northwestern University, where he remained as assistant and associate professor of neuropathology until 1944. At the invitation of George B. Hassin, he was one of the founders of the *Journal of Neuropathology and Experimental Neurology*, and it was at his insistence that "Experimental Neurology" was incorporated into the title. He was on the editorial board of the *Journal* from 1942 to 1950, associate editor from 1951 to 1952, coeditor from 1953 to 1961, and editor from 1962 until his retirement in 1963. His research interests covered all aspects of neuropathology and its related fields.

Louise Eisenhardt (1891–1967) was born in Ramsey, New Jersey (32). In 1915 she entered Harvey Cushing's office as an editorial assistant and worked with him on the book *Tumors of the Nervus Acousticus*. After he left for military duty in France she completed the work on the book, prepared the index, and saw it through the press. Deciding to obtain a medical education she entered Tufts Medical School, graduating in 1925 with the highest record ever obtained at Tufts. She interned at the Boston Hospital for Women and then was appointed neuropathologist under Cushing's direction at the Peter Bent Brigham Hospital, although she continued to take courses in neuropathology at Tufts. When Cushing went to Yale University in 1933 she stayed in Boston to complete the Brain Tumor Registry, taking it to New Haven with her in 1934. In 1943, when the Harvey Cushing Society established the *Journal of Neurosurgery*, she was made managing editor. The first issue of the *Journal* appeared in January 1944. Her death ended a career of service to neurosurgery, neuropathology, and the editorial arts.

Cyril Brian Courville (1900–1968) was born in Traverse City, Michigan. After graduating from Andrews University in Michigan, he entered the College of Medical Evangelists (now the Loma Linda University School of Medicine) from which he was graduated in 1925. He spent the year 1927 to 1928 as a voluntary assistant to Harvey Cushing, and it was at that time that he became interested in neuropathology. He served as a resident in neurosurgery and neurology at the Los Angeles County General Hospital from 1928 to 1932, when he was appointed to the faculty of his alma mater and to the staff of the Los Angeles County General Hospital. Shortly thereafter he was made professor of nervous diseases at Loma Linda. With the opening of the new county hospital in 1934 he established the Santiago Ramon y Cajal Laboratory of Neuropathology there. He was skilled in freehand drawing, and his popular lectures were illustrated by excellent sketches. With Johannes Nielsen and Carl Rand he established the Los Angeles Neurological Society and its *Bulletin*. He was best known for his important studies on cerebral trauma and anoxia carried out on the enormous pathologic material of the Los Angeles County General Hospital (14,15).

Neurosurgeons

Ernest Sachs (1879–1958) was graduated from Harvard University in 1900 and from The Johns Hopkins Medical School in 1904, following which he spent 3 years in residency at Mount Sinai Hospital (31). He was interested in neurosurgery, and his uncle Bernard Sachs arranged for him to work with Victor Horsley in London following a 6-month interval in Berlin where he studied neurology in Oppenheim's clinic. He spent his first months in London as a clinical clerk at the National Hospital in the morning and doing experimental work in Horsley's laboratory at University College in the afternoon. It was at University College that he completed his paper "On the Structure and Functional Relations of the Optic Thalamus," which appeared in *Brain* in 1909 (64). He accepted an invitation to develop neurosurgery at the newly organized Washington University Medical School in St. Louis, and became the world's first professor of neurosurgery. His publications were many, and through his influence Washington University became an important training center for neurology and neurosurgery.

Howard Christian Naffziger (1884–1961), born in California (69), received his bachelor's degree from the University of California in Berkeley and his medical degree from the University of California in San Francisco. He followed this with surgical training at The Johns Hopkins Hospital under William Halstead and his then associate Harvey Cushing. In 1929 Naffziger was made professor and chairman of the department of surgery at the University of California in San Francisco but resigned in 1947 to head the first department of neurologic surgery at the University of California. He organized the first formal surgical training program west of the Mississippi River and the first neurosurgical training program west of the Rocky Mountains. He retired from the faculty in 1951 and served as a regent of the University of California from 1952 until his death. Among his contributions to neurosurgery were studies on trauma to the nervous system, analyses of spinal cord injuries, and development of peripheral nerve surgery. He also wrote on the circulation of the CSF, increased intracranial pressure, and altered spinal cord physiology.

Max Minor Peet (1885–1949), born in Michigan, graduated from the University of Michigan with a bachelor's degree in 1906 and a medical degree in 1910 (39). After a 2-year internship at the Rhode Island General Hospital, he went to the University of Pennsylvania as Robert Robinson Porter Fellow in Research Medicine. He remained there to train in neurosurgery under Charles Frazier and was also closely associated with William Spiller. He then returned to the University of Michigan, where he later became professor of surgery and chief of the section of neurosurgery. Peet was a skilled technician. He perfected Frazier's operation for trigeminal neuralgia by stripping the sensory root of the trigeminal nerve from the gasserian ganglion rather than excising the ganglion. He obtained higher levels of analgesia following anterolateral cordotomy by extending the incision of the spinal cord directly forward through the anterior root. In 1933 he performed his first bilateral splanchnic nerve resection for the treatment of essential hypertension and subsequently became well known for this procedure.

Starting in his youth, Peet was also an ornithologist. He was one of the early discoverers of the nesting place of the Kirtland warbler, and his specimens of this bird are in the American Museum of Natural History and the Smithsonian Institution. He had an immense collection of personally prepared specimens which he gave to the Museum of Natural History of the University of Michigan. Peet claimed that his proficiency acquired in surgery started with his preparation of a collection of hummingbird skins.

Alfred Washington Adson (1887–1951), born in Iowa (16), received his bachelor's degree from the University of Nebraska and his medical degree from the University of Pennsylvania in 1916. He then received an appointment as a fellow in general surgery at what was to become the Mayo Foundation in Rochester, Minnesota. He was appointed to the surgical staff of the Mayo Clinic in 1917. His early successful experience with five patients who had surgically amenable lesions of either the brain or the spinal cord led him to turn his interests to neurosurgery. Shortly thereafter, at the suggestion of William Mayo, he gave up general surgery and concentrated on neurosurgery. From 1921 until 1946 he was professor of neurosurgery in the Mayo Foundation and head of the section of neurosurgery in the Mayo Clinic, and in 1946 he became senior neurosurgeon. Among his interests were the surgical treatment of trigeminal neuralgia, cervical ribs in their relation to brachial plexus compression, and surgery of the sympathetic nervous system. He believed that the procedure of choice in the treatment of essential hypertension was surgical ablation of the entire celiac ganglion. He was a founder of the American Board of Neurological Surgery and remained a member until his death, at which time he was chairman of the board.

Wilder Graves Penfield (1891–1977) (Fig. 30) graduated from Princeton University, following which he studied at Oxford University as a Rhodes Scholar (5). He graduated from The Johns Hopkins Medical School in 1918. He decided early in his medical education to make neurology and neurosurgery, and especially the cure of epilepsy, his life work, and he followed this course successfully. He considered himself a neurologist as well as a neurosurgeon, and he thought these subjects should be taught and practiced together. His training was not orthodox but it was catholic. He studied neurophysiology under Charles Sherrington, neurology under Gordon Holmes and his associates, and neurosurgery under Cushing and Horsley. He learned silver staining and neuropathology under Pio del Rio Hortega in Madrid and the surgical treatment of epilepsy under Otfrid Foerster in Breslau. He was appointed to the faculty of the College of Physicians and Surgeons and the staff of Presbyterian Hospital in New York City, and he established a laboratory of neurocytology at the Presbyterian Hospital. His accomplishments came to the attention of Alan Gregg, director of

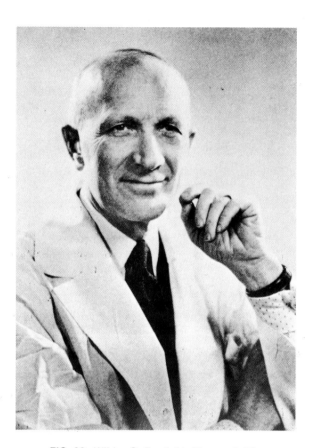

FIG. 30. Wilder G. Penfield. (From ref. 5.)

medical sciences and vice president of the Rockefeller Foundation. Through Gregg's influence, the Rockefeller Foundation supported the building of the Montreal Neurological Institute at McGill University. With Penfield as its director, the Institute soon became one of the leading training centers in neurology, neurosurgery, neurophysiology, and allied sciences. Penfield's major interest was the surgical treatment of epilepsy, but his concepts and contributions covered all aspects of brain function and disorders of function (53,54). He was author or co-author of a large number of important papers, monographs, and books on cerebral localization. During his later years he also wrote on historical, cultural, and sociologic subjects and even wrote some fiction (55). His autobiography appeared posthumously in 1977 (56).

REFERENCES

1. Adams, R. D. (1975): Stanley Cobb 1887–1968. In: *Centennial Anniversary Volume of the American Neurological Association 1875–1975,* edited by D. Denny-Brown, A. S. Rose, and A. L. Sahs, pp. 253–259. Springer, New York.

2. Ariëns Kappers, C. U., Huber, G. C., and Crosby, E. C. (1936): *The Comparative Anatomy of the Nervous System of Vertebrates, Including Man,* Vol. 2. Macmillan, New York.
3. Bard, P. (1970): Joseph Erlanger (1874–1965). In: *The Founders of Neurology,* 2nd Ed., edited by W. Haymaker and F. Schiller, pp. 190–195. Charles C Thomas, Springfield, Illinois.
4. Berger, H. (1929): Über das Elektroenkephalogram des Menschen. *Arch. Psychiatr.,* 87:527–535.
5. Boldrey, E. B. (1975): Wilder Graves Penfield 1891– . In: *Centennial Anniversary Volume of the American Neurological Association 1875–1975,* edited by D. Denny-Brown, A. S. Rose, and A. L. Sahs, pp. 263–269. Springer, New York.
6. Brazier, M. A. B. (1961): *A History of the Electrical Activity of the Brain: The First Century.* Macmillan, New York.
7. Bucy, P. C. (1975): Roland Parks Mackay 1900–1968. In: *Centennial Anniversary Volume of the American Neurological Association 1875–1975,* edited by D. Denny-Brown, A. S. Rose, and A. L. Sahs, pp. 277–280. Springer, New York.
8. Bucy, P. C. (1975): Percival Bailey 1892–1973. In: *Centennial Anniversary Volume of the American Neurological Association 1875–1975,* edited by D. Denny-Brown, A. S. Rose, and A. L. Sahs, pp. 280–284. Springer, New York.
9. Bucy, P. C. (1960): John Farquhar Fulton 1899–1960. *Arch. Neurol.,* 3:606–609.
10. Campbell, B. (1956): Andrew T. Rasmussen 1883–1954. *Trans. Am. Neurol. Assoc.,* 81:191–192.
11. Carter, S. (1975): Hiram Houston Merritt 1902–1978. In: *Centennial Anniversary Volume of the American Neurological Association 1875–1975,* edited by D. Denny-Brown, A. S. Rose, and A. L. Sahs, pp. 289–293. Springer, New York.
12. Castle, W. F. (1929): Observations on etiologic relationship of achylia gastrica to pernicious anemia. *Am. J. Med. Sci.,* 178:148–152.
13. Cobb, S. (1961): William Gordon Lennox, M.D. 1884–1960. *Arch. Neurol.,* 4:453–466.
14. Courville, C. B. (1953): *Commotio Cerebri: Cerebral Concussion and the Postconcussion Syndrome in Their Medical Legal Aspects.* Los Angeles, San Lucas Press.
15. Courville, C. B. (1967): Intracranial tumors: notes upon three thousand verified with some current observations pertaining to their mortality. *Bull. Los Angeles Neurol. Soc.,* 32:1–80.
16. Craig, W. McK. (1952): Alfred Washington Adson—Pioneer neurosurgeon 1887–1951. *J. Neurosurg.,* 9:117–123.
17. Crosby, E. C., Humphrey, T., and Lauer, E. W. (1962): *Correlative Anatomy of the Nervous System.* Macmillan, New York.
18. Davis, L. (1975): Lewis John Pollock 1886–1966. In: *Centennial Anniversary Volume of the American Neurological Association 1875–1975,* edited by D. Denny-Brown, A. S. Rose, and A. L. Sahs, pp. 232–236. Springer, New York.
19. Denny-Brown, D. (1975): James Bourne Ayer 1882–1963. In: *Centennial Anniversary Volume of the American Neurological Association 1875–1975,* edited by D. Denny-Brown, A. S. Rose, and A. L. Sahs. Springer, New York.
20. Dow, R. S. (1964): Olof Larsell 1885–1960. *Trans. Am. Neurol. Assoc.,* 89:982–983.
21. Ecker, A., and Riemenschneider, F. A. (1955): *Angiographic Localization of Intracranial Masses.* Charles C Thomas, Springfield, Illinois.
22. Everett, C. M., and Richards, R. K. (1944): Comparative anticonvulsive action of 5,5,5 trimethyloxazolidine 2,4 dione (tridione), Dilantin and phenobarbital. *J. Pharmacol. Exp. Ther.,* 31:402–419.
23. Ferraro, A. (1953): Joseph H. Globus 1885–1952. *J. Neuropathol. Exp. Neurol.,* 12:1–2.
24. Finley, K. H. (1975): Walter Frank Scheller 1879–1970. In: *Centennial Anniversary Volume of the American Neurological Association 1875–1975,* edited by D. Denny-Brown, A. S. Rose, and A. L. Sahs, pp. 242–246. Springer, New York.
25. Foley, J. M. (1975): Derek Ernest Denny-Brown 1901– . In: *Centennial Anniversary Volume of the American Neurological Association 1875–1975,* edited by D. Denny-Brown, A. S. Rose, and A. L. Sahs, pp. 301–308. Springer, New York.
26. Forster, F. M. (1975): Hans Heinrich Reese 1891–1973. In: *Centennial Anniversary Volume of the American Neurological Association 1875–1975,* edited by D. Denny-Brown, A. S. Rose, and A. L. Sahs, pp. 273–277. Springer, New York.

27. Fulton, J. F. (1943): *Physiology of the Nervous System.* Oxford University Press, New York.
28. Fulton, J. F. (1946): *Harvey Cushing: A Biography.* Charles C Thomas, Springfield, Illinois.
29. Fulton, J. F. (1951): *Frontal Lobotomy and Affective Behavior: A Neurophysiological Analysis.* W. W. Horton, New York.
30. Fulton, J. F. (1970): Johannes Gregorius Dusser de Barenne. In: *The Founders of Neurology,* 2nd Ed., edited by W. Haymaker and F. Schiller, pp. 186–190. Charles C Thomas, Springfield, Illinois.
31. Furlow, L. T., and O'Leary, J. L. (1975): Ernest Sachs 1879–1958. In: *Centennial Anniversary Volume of the American Neurological Association 1875–1975,* edited by D. Denny-Brown, A. S. Rose, and A. L. Sahs, pp. 236–239. Springer, New York.
32. German, W. J. (1967): Louise Eisenhardt 1891–1967. *Trans. Am. Neurol. Assoc.,* 92:311–313.
33. Gerty, F. J. (1975): Harold Douglas Singer 1875–1940. In: *Centennial Anniversary Volume of the American Neurological Association 1875–1975,* edited by D. Denny-Brown, A. S. Rose, and A. L. Sahs, pp. 224–228. Springer, New York.
34. Globus, J. (1952): George B. Hassin, M.D. *J. Neuropathol. Exp. Neurol.,* 11:1–3.
35. Goodell, H., and Plum, F. (1975): Harold George Wolff 1898–1962. In: *Centennial Anniversary Volume of the American Neurological Association 1875–1975,* edited by D. Denny-Brown, A. S. Rose, and A. L. Sahs, pp. 308–313. Springer, New York.
36. Haymaker, W.: James Papez (1883–1958). In: *The Founders of Neurology,* 2nd Ed., edited by W. Haymaker and F. Schiller, pp. 143–147. Charles C Thomas, Springfield, Illinois.
37. Hinsey, J. D. (1970): Herbert Gasser (1888–1963). In: *The Founders of Neurology,* 2nd Ed., edited by W. Haymaker and F. Schiller, pp. 213–217. Charles C Thomas, Springfield, Illinois.
38. Huber, C. P. (1936): Gotthelf Carl Huber, biographical sketch. In: *G. Carl Huber Memorial Volume,* pp. 1–3. Wistar Institute, Philadelphia.
39. Kahn, E. A. (1976): Max Minor Peet 1885–1949. *Surg. Neurol.,* 3:65–69.
40. Larsell, O. (1951): *The Cerebellum: A Review and Interpretation.* Appleton-Century-Crofts, New York.
41. Larsell, O. (1970): George Coghill (1873–1941). In: *The Founders of Neurology,* 2nd Ed., edited by W. Haymaker and F. Schiller, pp. 104–106. Charles C Thomas, Springfield, Illinois.
42. Levy, I. (1975): James Lee O'Leary 1904–   . In: *Centennial Anniversary Volume of the American Neurological Association 1875–1975,* edited by D. Denny-Brown, A. S. Rose, and A. L. Sahs, pp. 313–318. Springer, New York.
43. Magoun, H. W.: Stephen Ransom (1880–1942). In: *The Founders of Neurology,* 2nd Ed., edited by W. Haymaker and F. Schiller, pp. 152–154. Charles C Thomas, Springfield, Illinois.
44. McHenry, L. C., Jr. (1975): William Biddle Cadwalader (1876–1957). In: *Centennial Anniversary Volume of the American Neurological Association 1875–1975,* edited by D. Denny-Brown, A. S. Rose, and A. L. Sahs, pp. 216–219. Springer, New York.
46. Merritt, H. H. (1975): Samuel Bernard Wortis 1904–1959. In: *Centennial Anniversary Volume of the American Neurological Association 1875–1975,* edited by D. Denny-Brown, A. S. Rose, and A. L. Sahs, pp. 246–250. Springer, New York.
46. Merritt, H. H. (1975): Samual Bernard Wortis 1904–1959. In: *Centennial Anniversary Volume of the American Neurological Association 1875–1975,* edited by D. Denny-Brown, A. S. Rose, and A. L. Sahs, pp. 269–272. Springer, New York.
47. Minot, G. H., and Murphy, W. P. (1926): Treatment of pernicious anemia by special diet. *J.A.M.A.,* 87:470–472.
48. Mixter, W. J., and Barr, J. S. (1934): Rupture of intervertebral disc with involvement of spinal cord. *N. Engl. J. Med.,* 211:210–212.
49. Moniz, E. (1927): L'encephalographie arteriélle son importance dans le localization des tumeurs cerébrales. *Rev. Neurol. (Paris),* 2:72–90.
50. Moore, J. B., Jr. (1963): Epidemiology of syphilis. *J.A.M.A.,* 186:831–835.
51. Mulder, D. W. (1975): Henry William Woltman 1889–1964. In: *Centennial Anniversary Volume of the American Neurological Association 1875–1975,* edited by D. Denny-Brown, A. S. Rose, and A. L. Sahs, pp. 259–263. Springer, New York.

52. Papez, J. W. (1937): A proposed mechanism of emotions. *Arch. Neurol. Psychiatry,* 38:725–743.
53. Penfield, W., and Jasper, H. (1954): *Epilepsy and the Functional Anatomy of the Brain.* Little, Brown, Boston.
54. Penfield, W., and Rasmussen, T. (1951): *The Cerebral Cortex of Man.* Macmillan, New York.
55. Penfield, W. (1960): *The Torch.* Little, Brown, Boston.
56. Penfield, W. (1977): *No Man Alone: A Neurosurgeon's Life.* Little, Brown, Boston.
57. Ransom, S. E. (1920): *The Anatomy of the Nervous System.* Saunders, Philadelphia.
58. Rasmussen, A. T. (1932): *The Principal Nervous Pathways.* Macmillan, New York.
59. Richardson, J. C. (1950): Some recent changes in clinical neurology. *Can. Med. Assoc. J.,* 83:432–436.
60. Richter, R. B. (1970): In memorium: Arthur Weil 1887–1969. *J. Neuropathol. Exp. Neurol.,* 29:1–5.
61. Rickes, E. I., Brink, N. G., Koniussy, F. B., et al. (1958): Crystalline vitamin B$_{12}$. *Science,* 107:396–400.
62. Rudnick, D.: Ross Harrison (1870–1959). In: *The Founders of Neurology,* 2nd Ed., edited by W. Haymaker and F. Schiller, pp. 104–107. Charles C Thomas, Springfield, Illinois.
63. Sabin, A. B. (1959): Status of field trials with orally administered live attenuated poliomyelitis vaccine. *J.A.M.A.,* 171:265–267.
64. Sachs, E. (1909): On the structure and functional relations of the optic thalamus. *Brain,* 32:95–186.
65. Salk, J. (1955): Contribution to preparation and use of poliomyelitis virus vaccine. *J.A.M.A.,* 158:1239–1241.
66. Schwab, R. S. (1970): Obituary: Henry R. Viets, M.D. 1890–1969. *Arch. Neurol.,* 23:187–188.
67. Shulman, S. (1975): Richard Biddle Richter 1901–1971. In: *Centennial Anniversary Volume of the American Neurological Association 1875–1975,* edited by D. Denny-Brown, A. S. Rose, and A. L. Sahs, pp. 322–327. Springer, New York.
68. Sprofkin, D. E. (1961): Sam Lillard Clark 1896–1960. *Trans Am. Neurol. Assoc.,* 86:262.
69. Stern, W. E. (1961): Howard Christian Naffziger 1884–1961. *J. Neurosurg.,* 15:711–713.
70. Symonds, C. P. (1923): Contribution to clinical study of intracranial aneurysms. *Guys Hosp. Rep.,* 73:139–159.
71. Victor, M. (1958): Alcohol and nutritional disease of the nervous system. *J.A.M.A.,* 197:85–87.
72. Von Hagen, K. O. (1975): Johannes Maagaard Nielsen 1890–1969. In: *Centennial Anniversary Volume of the American Neurological Association 1875–1975,* edited by D. Denny-Brown, A. S. Rose, and A. L. Sahs, pp. 284–289. Springer, New York.
73. Wegeforth, F., Ayer, J. B., and Essick, C. R. (1919): The method of obtaining cerebrospinal fluid by puncture of the cisterna magna (cistern puncture). *Am. J. Med. Sci.,* 157:789–797.
74. Weibel, J., and Fields, W. S. (1968): *Atlas of Arteriography of Occlusive Cerebrovascular Disease.* Saunders, Philadelphia.
75. Weinstein, E. A. (1975): Israel Strauss 1873–1955. In: *Centennial Anniversary Volume of the American Neurological Association 1875–1975,* edited by D. Denny-Brown, A. S. Rose, and A. L. Sahs, pp. 195–198. Springer, New York.
76. Weinstein, E. A. (1975): Israel Spanier Wechsler 1886–1962. In: *Centennial Anniversary Volume of the American Neurological Association 1875–1975,* edited by D. Denny-Brown, A. S. Rose, and A. L. Sahs, pp. 293–296. Springer, New York.
77. Wolff, H. G. (1946): *Headache and Other Head Pain.* Oxford University Press, New York.

7

American Board of Psychiatry and Neurology

Specialization in medical practice developed during the latter decades of the last half of the nineteenth century and rapidly progressed during the early decades of the twentieth. There was much concern, however, on the part of many physicians that there were no criteria for assessing adequacy of training in the various specialties and no yardstick for measuring professional competence. Membership or fellowship in some of the more prestigious specialty societies or colleges was an indirect recognition of such training and competence, and this was used for specialty recognition in several European countries. However, the criteria for such membership varied from one society to another, and no uniform standards were available (8).

In 1920 the Council on Medical Education and Hospitals of the American Medical Association (AMA) appointed committees in the various medical specialties which were asked to recommend the training necessary in each specialty that would qualify the physician as an expert in that field. The Council had published the first list of approved internships in 1914, at which time 95 hospitals were listed as offering training in some specialized field of medicine. In 1927 the Council published the first list of hospitals specifically approved by it for residency in the various specialties. There were 699 approved residencies in 270 hospitals (7).

The first board of certification of a medical specialty in the United States was the American Board of Ophthalmology, which was organized in 1916. The American Board of Otolaryngology was established in 1924, the American Board of Obstetrics and Gynecology in 1930, and the American Board of Dermatology in 1932 (7,8).

Adolph Meyer's presidential address to the American Psychiatric Association at its annual meeting in 1928 recommended that the various centers in which psychiatric training was carried out develop intensive training courses, at the completion of which diplomas could be issued (11). In an editorial in the *American Journal of Psychiatry* in 1931, Franklin G. Ebaugh advocated the formation of an American board of examiners in psychiatry

(6). Also in 1931, the Section on Nervous and Mental Disease of the AMA acknowledged the need for adopting standards of training and certification in psychiatry and neurology, and resolved "active cooperation in this educational movement."

At the meeting of the American Psychiatric Association in Boston in May 1933, a Board of Examiners was appointed (13), comprising Clarence O. Cheney (chairman), Aldof Meyer, William A. White, C. Macfie Campbell, and Franklin G. Ebaugh. The Section on Nervous and Mental Disease of the AMA met the next month in Milwaukee, and at that meeting it was proposed that the Section cooperate with other concerned national organizations for the purpose of establishing an examining board in psychiatry and neurology (7). A committee consisting of Walter Freeman (chairman), Lloyd H. Ziegler, Edwin G. Zabriskie, J. Allen Jackson, and George W. Hall was appointed to implement this. The American Neurological Association later that same month appointed a similar committee consisting of J. Ramsey Hunt, Israel S. Wechsler, and Henry A. Riley to work with the other committees (12).

Members of the three committees met together to discuss training requirements and examination procedures. The philosophies of each discipline were reviewed, and there was controversy over which should be dominant. The representatives from the American Psychiatric Association expressed the opinion that orientation be primarily toward psychiatry, those from the American Neurological Association stressed neurology, whereas those from the AMA's Section on Nervous and Mental Disease believed that the ultimate goal should be toward the training and certification of neuropsychiatrists. It was finally decided that a board should be appointed which had equal representation from all three organizations, with four members appointed by the American Psychiatric Association, four by the American Neurological Association, and four (two psychiatrists and two neurologists) by the AMA's Section on Nervous and Mental Disease. There would be separate qualifications, examinations, and certification for psychiatry and neurology, and candidates who wished certification in both would have to pass examinations in each.

The first American Board of Psychiatry and Neurology was appointed in 1934, with the following members: from the American Psychiatric Association, Meyer, Cheney, Campbell, and Ebaugh; from the American Neurological Association, Zabriskie, Louis Casamajor, Lewis J. Pollock, and H. Douglas Singer; from the Section on Nervous and Mental Disease, Hall, Jackson, Freeman, and Ziegler (Fig. 31). The first meeting was held on October 20, 1934, in New York, with Meyer acting as chairman. Singer was elected president, Campbell vice-president, and Freeman secretary-treasurer. The Board had been incorporated in Wilmington, Delaware, the previous day, and the appointees were named directors of the corporation. There was much discussion about the priority of specialties in the name of

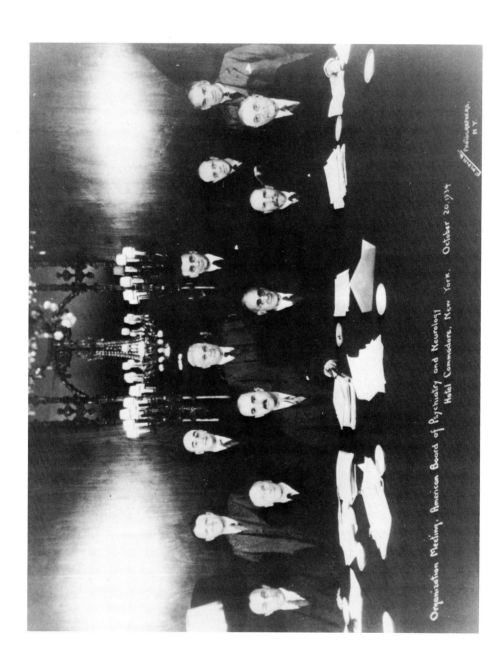

Organization Meeting, American Board of Psychiatry and Neurology, Hotel Commodore, New York. October 20, 1934

the board, and it was decided to place the term psychiatry first because of the numerical consituency of those to be examined by the Board. Casamajor was "unable to understand the alphabetical ignorance of this" (7).

It was decided that there should be a "grandfather clause" under which those already practicing the specialties could be certified without examination. Accordingly, it was decreed that those physicians who had graduated from medical school in 1919 or before and had carried on specialized practice for 15 years could be certified without examination. Those who had graduated between 1919 and 1929 and had practiced 5 years or less were required to pass the examination for certification. Those who had graduated between 1929 and 1934 had to show evidence that they had adequate training and experience and in addition were required to pass the examination. Those who had graduated after 1934 were required to serve an internship as well as 3 years of training in an institution approved for training in the specialty by the Council on Medical Education and Hospitals of the AMA, followed by 2 years of specialized practice, and then to pass the examination. The first examinations given by the Board were held at the Philadelphia General Hospital on June 7 and 8, 1934.

Singer served as president of the Board from 1934 until his death in 1940, after which presidents were elected annually from the membership of the Board. Freeman served as secretary-treasurer through 1946, when he was succeeded by Francis J. Braceland, who served from 1947 through 1951. He in turn was succeeded by David A. Boyd Jr., who served in this capacity through his term as an elected member of the Board, following which he was appointed executive secretary-treasurer, serving in this capacity until 1971. Russell N. DeJong served as interim executive secretary-treasurer for 1 year (1971–1972), when Lester H. Rudy was appointed executive secretary-treasurer. In 1974 the title was changed to that of executive director.

During the years changes have been made in the conduct and content of the examination. In 1959, recognizing that child psychiatry was a specific field of subspecialization in psychiatry, the American Board of Psychiatry and Neurology, with the concurrence of the Advisory Board of Medical Specialties, established a Committee on Certification in Child Psychiatry. This Committee issues certificates of specialization in child psychiatry, operating under the supervision of and in accordance with the policies of the Board. It consists of six members certified in child psychiatry by the Committee and one member certified in pediatrics by the American Board of Pediatrics. In 1968 the Board acknowledged that pediatric neurology was an important subspecialty by issuing certificates in neurology with special competence in child neurology as well as those in general neurology.

FIG. 31. The first American Board of Psychiatry and Neurology. *First row:* Cheney, Campbell, Freeman, Singer, Meyer, Hall. *Second row:* Ebaugh, Casamajor, Jackson, Ziegler, Pollock, Zabriskie. (Courtesy of Lester H. Rudy.)

For a period of 2 years, from December 1965 through 1967, written as well as oral examinations were given in basic neurology and basic psychiatry, "not to replace any part of the oral examination, but in addition to it." It was hoped that the experience gained from evaluation of this concomitant written test would aid in planning an effective written screening test. Starting in 1968, the examination in the basic subjects was given as a written test and the oral examination was eliminated. Shortly thereafter the use of photographs and X-rays was incorporated into the written test, and in 1977 the use of audiovisual case presentations was substituted for some of the living patient presentations.

During the early 1970s most of the medical specialty boards dropped the requirement of serving an internship prior to entering a residency training program, and the American Board of Psychiatry and Neurology did so in 1973. General dissatisfaction about this, however, especially on the part of the neurologists, led to the establishment in 1974 of a "clinical experience first year" during which, prior to entering a residency training program, the medical school graduate would be required to have a year of clinical experience with special emphasis on internal medicine, pediatrics, or family practice. This could be obtained either in a categorical internship or as the first year of a 4-year residency training program.

In 1975 the Board was enlarged to 16 members in order to allow more organizations to have representation on it. Membership was determined to be as follows: five from the American Psychiatric Association, three from the Section Council on Psychiatry of the AMA, four from the American Neurological Association, and two each from the American Academy of Neurology and the Section Council on Neurology of the AMA.

Beginning in 1973 the subject of recertification was discussed, and committees were appointed to make plans for instituting it. The subject was still under discussion in 1980.

Among the first obligations of the American Board of Psychiatry and Neurology were establishing criteria for training and determining which training programs gave satisfactory graded training (2,8). These were done separately for psychiatry and neurology. Residency Review Committees were appointed in each specialty, with half of the members of the Committee also members of the Board, and half of the members appointed by the Council on Medical Education and Hospitals of the AMA. Eventually each training program was reviewed every 3 years, and a decision was made to approve it for 1, 2, or 3 years of training. Thirteen programs were approved for training in neurology in 1934 (9), and 22 programs in 1940 (10). In 1950, 69 programs were approved for the training of 209 residents (1). In 1960, 85 programs were approved for 3 years of training for 378 residents, 29 programs were approved for 2 years of training of 42 residents, and 17 were approved for 1 year of training of 34 residents (3). In 1970, 88 programs were approved for 3 years of training of 331 residents, two were approved for 2 years of training of three residents, and four were approved for 1 year of training of 12 residents (4). In 1980 a total of 125 programs was approved for training in neurology (5).

REFERENCES

1. (1950): Approved internships and residencies in the United States and Canada. *J.A.M.A.*, 142:1179.
2. Curran, J. H. (1959): Internships and residencies: Historical background and current trends. *J. Med. Educ.*, 34:873−884.
3. (1960): Directory of approved residencies. *J.A.M.A.*, 174:707−709.
4. (1970): *Directory of Approved Internships and Residencies*, pp. 177−182. American Medical Association, Chicago.
5. (1980): *Directory of Approved Internships and Residencies*, pp. 129−136. American Medical Association, Chicago.
6. Ebaugh, F. G. (1931): Editorial. *Am. J. Psychiatry*, 10:873.
7. Freeman, W. A., Ebaugh, F. G., and Boyd, D. A., Jr. (1959): The founding of the American Board of Psychiatry and Neurology. *Am. J. Psychiatry*, 115:769−778.
8. Johnson, V. (1962): The historical development of accreditation in medical education. *J.A.M.A.*, 181:616−619.
9. (1934): Medical education in the United States and Canada. *J.A.M.A.*, 103:599.
10. (1940): Medical education in the United States and Canada. *J.A.M.A.*, 115:768.
11. Meyer, A. (1928−1929): Presidential address: Twenty-five years of psychiatry in the United States and our present outlook. *Am. J. Psychiatry*, 8:1−31.
12. (1930−1931): Notes and comments: the suggested American board of examiners in psychiatry. *Am. J. Psychiatry*, 10:873−876.
13. Rudy, L. H. (1980): American Board of Psychiatry and Neurology. In: *Comprehensive Textbook of Psychiatry*, 3rd Ed., edited by A. M. Freedman and H. I. Kaplan, pp. 135−147. Williams and Wilkins, Baltimore.

8

American Academy of Neurology

Following World War II there was rapid expansion of American neurology. Antibiotics and advances in pharmacotherapy were making treatment procedures available for many neurologic disorders. Pneumoencephalography, electroencephalography, innovations in the cerebrospinal fluid examination, and, more recently, angiography were contributing to more accurate and reliable diagnoses; and refinements in surgical techniques were making neurosurgery more safe and predictable. Experience during and after World War II was showing that neurology could and should be practiced as a separate specialty. As a consequence, many young physicians were becoming interested in the field and were seeking opportunities for training. The American Board of Psychiatry and Neurology had been organized, and increasing numbers of training programs in the neurologic sciences were being approved by the Board and by the Council on Medical Education and Hospitals of the American Medical Association (AMA). However, medical educators throughout the country were aware that these programs needed improvement and enlargement, and that there was an increasing demand for well-trained neurologists.

It became apparent to many who were entering the specialty that there were no medical societies in the United States devoted exclusively to neurology in which neophytes in the field could participate. There was no organization in which young neurologists and residents could meet and talk with their more mature colleagues. The American Neurological Association had been in existence since 1875, but its membership was limited to senior neurologists; those wishing to be considered for membership were required to have written a number of published papers and, in addition, to write a thesis which would be critically reviewed. The AMA's Section on Nervous and Mental Disease included neurologists and psychiatrists, and its meetings were poorly attended. The meetings of the Association for Research in Nervous and Mental Disease were well attended, but its members met close to the Christmas season and its meeting dealt with the research aspects of a single subject, which might be either psychiatric or neurologic.

In 1947 a resident in the neurology training program at the University of

Minnesota, Joseph A. Resch (currently chairman of the department there), called the situation to the attention of his chief, Abe B. Baker. Recognizing the need for an organization for the younger men in the specialty, Baker launched plans to create a new national neurologic society with a relatively unrestricted membership. In October 1947 he sent a letter to more than 50 of the leading American teachers, clinicians, and investigators in the neurologic sciences, seeking their opinions regarding the need and desire for such an organization. The response to the letter was enthusiastic, and the replies were almost unanimously in favor of the idea. Thus the American Academy of Neurology was born. Those responding to the letter became the charter members of the Academy and were named the first 52 Fellows of the Academy; these included: Raymond D. Adams, Robert B. Aird, Bernard J. Alpers, Pearce Bailey, Abe B. Baker, Clemens E. Benda, Benjamin B. Boshes, Joe R. Brown, Walter L. Bruetsch, Derek Denny-Brown (who soon resigned), Cyril B. Courville, C. G. de Guitierrez-Mahoney, Russell N. De-Jong, Lee H. Eaton, Francis M. Forster, Sherman F. Gilpin Jr., Robert W. Graves, Webb Haymaker, Paul F. A. Hoefer, Walter O. Klingman, Lawrence C. Kolb, O. R. Langworthy, Frederic H. Lewey, Benjamin W. Lichtenstein, Samuel C. Little, Wilmot S. Litteljohn, Roland P. Mackay, H. Houston Merritt, Frederick P. Moersch, Johannes M. Nielsen, Harold H. Noran, Richard B. Richter, Adolph L. Sahs, Manuel Saul, Walter F. Schaller, Nathan E. Schlesinger, Robert S. Schwab, Gabriel A. Schwarz, John E. Skogland, William A. Smith, Theodore L. L. Soniat, A. Theodore Steegman, Winifred Bayard Stewart, Theodore T. Stone, George H. Thompson, Carroll C. Turner, Henry H. Viets, Karl O. Von Hagen, Robert Wartenberg, Richard Wilson, Henry W. Woltman, and Paul Yakovlev.

The American Academy of Neurology was incorporated in Minnesota on March 13, 1948, with Aird, Forster, and Baker as witnesses. An organizational meeting was held in Chicago on June 23, 1948, at the time of the AMA meeting, with an attendance of more than 50. The following officers were elected: president, Abe B. Baker; vice-president, Pearce Bailey; secretary-treasurer, Joe R. Brown. These men were to serve as interim officers for 1 year and then hold office for 2 years.

The first scientific meeting of the Academy was held at French Lick Springs, Indiana, in June 1949, with Dave B. Ruskin serving as program chairman. At this time a Board of Trustees consisting of Frederic H. Lewey, Johannes N. Nielsen, Adolph L. Sahs, and William A. Smith was elected. Thirty-eight papers were presented during the 3-day meeting.

From the beginning the Academy had several categories of membership. Active membership requires certification in neurology by the American Board of Psychiatry and Neurology; only active members are eligible to hold office. Creation of the junior membership provided the privilege of participating in scientific meetings by young members not yet certified as well as residents in training. There are two categories of associate membership:

Clinical associate members are practitioners of neurology who have acquired approved training but are not yet certified in neurology. Nonclinical associate members are those in allied fields—neuroanatomy, neuropathology, neurophysiology, etc.—but not clinical neurologists. Any active member who limits his or her practice to neurology and who has made significant contributions to neurologic education and the neurologic literature is eligible for election to fellowship.

The 1950 meeting of the American Academy of Neurology (at that time called the first interim meeting) was held in Cincinnati. Twenty-three scientific papers were read, and a symposium on psychomotor epilepsy was held. A highlight of the meeting was a talk on virus diseases of the nervous system by Albert Sabin. At this meeting, Pearce Bailey assumed the position of president-elect, and Howard D. Fabing was elected vice-president. The Board of Trustees authorized the publication of a new journal, to be called *Neurology,* which would be the official publication of the Academy, and Russell N. DeJong was made editor-in-chief. Also at this meeting the Woman's Auxiliary of the Academy was organized with Mrs. William N. Hughes as first president. The Auxiliary was to play an important role in the social activities of the Academy, and wives were encouraged to attend meetings with their husbands. After the Cincinnati meeting the American Academy of Neurology met annually during the last week in April, and the term ''interim meeting'' was no longer used.

By the time of the 1951 meeting of the Academy in Virginia Beach, Virginia, the membership in the Academy had grown to a total of 860. At this meeting 30 scientific papers were read, there were seven exhibits, and a special course in neuropathology was offered and was well received. At the meeting in Louisville in 1952, 22 papers were read, there were 12 exhibits, and a symposium on pediatric neurology was held. In addition, the special courses continued to be in demand and were well attended, and at this time courses in neuropathology, neuroradiology, and electroencephalography were presented. At the meeting in Chicago in 1953, 35 scientific papers were read, there were 22 scientific exhibits and eight commerical exhibits, and eight special courses were offered.

An annual lecture in honor of Robert Wartenberg, who had died the previous year, was instituted at the meeting of the American Academy of Neurology in Boston in 1957. The first Wartenberg Lecture was given by Gunnar Wohlfart of Lund, Sweden. During the next several years these Lectures were presented by the following: J. Godwin Greenfield of London, James W. F. Bull of London, Macdonald Critchley of London, Paul E. Polani of London, W. Ritchie Russell of Oxford, Sigvald Refsum of Oslo, Michael Kremer of London, Derek Denny-Brown of Boston, H. Houston Merritt of New York, George C. Cotzias of New York, Julius Axelrod of Bethesda, Paul Yakovlev of Boston, Abe B. Baker of Minneapolis, Mary A. B. Brazier of Los Angeles, Neal S. Miller of New York, Roger W. Gilliatt of London,

William H. Oldendorf of Los Angeles, John N. Walton of Newcastle upon Tyne, Henry J. M. Barnett of London, Ontario, and James Lance of Sydney, Australia.

An award named for S. Weir Mitchell was designed to stimulate an interest in basic and/or clinical investigation among junior members of the Academy. Each year junior members are encouraged to submit papers describing their research activities, and a committee is appointed to review the papers. The award is given annually to the person whose paper is judged to be the best of those submitted for the year, the recipient of the award is asked to read his paper at one of the scientific sessions of the annual meeting, and a monetary award and a medallion are presented to him by the Woman's Auxiliary. Many of the early awardees have maintained their interest in research and have risen to prominence in American neurology. The first S. Weir Mitchell Award was presented to John Logothetis in 1955, and during the next few years the following received the award: Ernst A. Rodin, D. Frank Benson, Wallace W. Tourellotte, Robert Katzman, Joel Brumlik, W. King Engel, Ture O. Tuncbay, Irwin A. Brody, Wigbert C. Wiederholt, John H. Seipel, Norman G. Bass, Peter C. Dowling and Stuart T. Cook (jointly), Margaret M. Waddington, Edwin H. Kolodny, Lorenz K. Y. Ng, Michael E. Goldberg, David Holtzman, Ronald M. Kobayashi, Howard Feit, Steven Novom, Robert W. Clark, Robert L. Macdonald, Lawrence Steinman, and Gavril Pasternak.

An essay award for medical students was developed during the 1960s. In the beginning guidelines were rather broad and nonspecific, but in 1971 three categories of awards were identified: A prize for an essay dealing with clinical neurology was named the G. Milton Shy Award; a prize for an essay dealing with experimental neurology was named the Saul R. Korey Award; and a prize for an essay dealing with general/historical aspects of neurology was called the Roland P. Mackay Award.

The annual meetings of the American Academy of Neurology are well and enthusiastically attended. The first 3 days of the week, Monday through Wednesday, are devoted to special courses, several being given simultaneously each day. Scientific sesssions and poster sessions are held on Thursday and Friday, and on Saturday morning. Business meetings follow the morning sessions on Thursday and Friday. Social gatherings and activities of the Auxiliary take place throughout the week. The Academy, through its many committees, has had significant influence on undergraduate medical education, neurologic training and certification, the practice of neurology, research in the neurologic sciences and clinical neurology, and national activities and legislation as related to medicine and neurology.

The Academy's presidents since its inception, each holding office for 2 years, have been the following: Abe B. Baker, Pearce Bailey, Howard D. Fabing, Walter O. Klingman, Francis M. Forster, Augustus S. Rose, Adolph L. Sahs, Joseph M. Foley, Charles A. Kane, Richard P. Schmidt, Sidney

Carter, Joe R. Brown, Gilbert H. Glaser, Robert A. Fishman, Robert J. Joynt, and Dewey H. Ziegler.

As of July 1979 there were 6,170 members in the American Academy of Neurology. Of these, 168 were senior members, 842 were fellows, 2,087 were active members, 1,644 were junior members, 946 were associate clinical members, 441 were associate nonclinical members, 11 were honorary members, and 31 were honorary-corresponding members.

9

Child Neurology Society

During the 1960s those neurologists who specialized in, or limited their practices to, the diagnosis and treatment of neurologic disorders affecting infants and children felt the need to establish their autonomy. To do this they believed it necessary to form a society that dealt primarily with the problems of child neurology, believing that such an organization would stimulate the development of scientific interest in the subspecialty and would contribute to the welfare of children with neurologic disorders. Such an organization became even more desirable in 1968 when the American Board of Psychiatry and Neurology established certification in child neurology by designating those qualified for it as certified in neurology with special competence in child neurology.

An organizational meeting of the proposed Child Neurology Society was held in La Crosse, Wisconsin, on November 26 and 27, 1971. It was attended by several midwestern child neurologists, mainly from academic institutions, who had strong feelings about the need for such an organization and believed it to be the first step toward the establishment of training fellowships in child neurology under the auspices of the National Institutes of Health. Those in attendance were Richard J. Allem, William S. Bell, Raymond W. M. Chun, Paul R. Dyken, Manuel R. Gomez, Kenneth F. Swaiman, George Wolcott, and Francis S. Wright. There was unanimous agreement that the founding of such a society was essential to the development of the discipline. It was decided to investigate the national feeling about such a move by circulating a questionnaire inquiring about the need for and interest in such a society which, if established, would meet annually for the presentation of papers dealing with neurologic disorders of infants and children and, incidentally, for the purpose of stimulating training in and expansion of the discipline. The response was positive, and a committee was appointed to proceed with plans for the first national scientific meeting to be held in Ann Arbor, Michigan, on October 5 to 7, 1972, with Swaiman serving as chairman.

The Ann Arbor meeting was well attended. The following officers were elected: president, Kenneth F. Swaiman; secretary-treasurer, Richard J.

Allen; counselors, Manuel R. Gomez, John H. Menkes, Isabelle Rapin, and James F. Schwartz. During the scientific sessions of the meeting 20 papers were presented, and in the business sessions committees were organized and future plans for the Society were formulated.

Since 1972 the Child Neurology Society has met annually and has grown in size and influence. The following have served as president: Gerald M. Fenichell (1973), Manuel R. Gomez (1974), James F. Schwartz (1975), Richard J. Allen (1976), Bruce D. Berg (1977), N. Paul Rosman (1978), Arthur L. Prensky (1979), Paul R. Dyken (1980), and Mary Ann Guggenheim (1981). The Child Neurology Society directory published in 1972 listed 25 members and 29 junior members; in 1980 there were 416 members and 84 junior members.

In 1974 the Akron Children's Hospital, through the efforts of G. Dean Timmons, established the Hower Award for the Society. Recipients have been as follows: Douglas N. Buchanan (1974), Randolph N. Byers (1975), Sidney Carter (1976), David B. Clark (1977), Philip R. Dodge (1978), Paul I. Yalovlev (1979), and John H. Menkes (1980).

In 1975 and 1976 negotiations were carried out between officers of the Child Neurology Society and the council of the American Neurological Association in regard to the establishment of a new neurologic journal, the *Annals of Neurology*. It was decided that it should be the official journal of the Child Neurology Society as well as the American Neurological Association, and the first issue of the *Annals of Neurology* was published in January 1977. The following members of the Child Neurology Society have served on its editorial board: Darryl C. DeVivo, Paul R. Dyken, Gerald D. Golden, and Kenneth F. Swaiman.

The Child Neurology Society has made significant contributions to the growth and development of American neurology by focusing attention on what had hitherto been a somewhat neglected aspect of it.

10

Neurologic Journals and Publications

Prior to 1900 most neurologic material, investigative and clinical, was published in either books or the general medical journals. The one exception was the *Journal of Nervous and Mental Disease,* which was first established during the 1870s and was still being published monthly over a century later. It preceded *Brain,* the major British neurologic journal, which first appeared in 1879, and the *Revue Neurologique,* which was not published until 1893. The other major American journals, the *Archives of Neurology, Neurology,* and the *Annals of Neurology,* did not appear until the twentieth century.

JOURNAL OF NERVOUS AND MENTAL DISEASE

The *Chicago Journal of Nervous and Mental Disease* was first issued as a quarterly publication in 1874 with James S. Jewell as editor and Henry M. Bannister as assistant editor. Two years later its title was changed to *Journal of Nervous and Mental Disease.* In the first issue Dr. Jewell stated, ''To discuss the nature, and, according to the best light we have, the practical management, of disorders of the nervous system, is one of the chief aims of the Editors in projecting their Journal. We do not believe that we mistake the feeling of many members of the profession, when we say they are looking for more information than is accessible to them, in regard to the nature and treatment of such diseases.'' Shortly after the founding of the American Neurological Association in 1875 the *Journal* became the official publication of the Association.

Jewell and Bannister remained as editors of the *Journal* for 8 years. In 1882 it was taken over by William G. Morton, who moved it to New York City; he served as editor for 4 years. In 1885 Bernard Sachs joined Morton as associate editor, and in 1886 he became proprietor of the *Journal* and succeeded Morton as editor. At this time the *Journal* was a monthly publication. Sachs served as editor during the years 1886 and 1887, then relinquished the position for financial reasons. In 1888 Graeme M. Hammond took over the *Journal* and became editor, and in 1889 Charles H. Brown joined him as associate editor. In 1890 Hammond also relinquished the *Journal* for financial reasons, and Brown assumed the responsibility for publication and became managing editor. In 1897 William G. Spiller was named associate editor, and in 1899 Spiller became editor and Smith Ely Jelliffe was named associate editor. Brown died in 1901, and Jelliffe purchased the *Journal* and became managing editor in 1902. Spiller served as editor-in-chief from 1902 to 1913, after which time Jelliffe served as managing editor without associates. Beginning in 1916 the *Journal* was published as two volumes each year. Jelliffe continued as managing editor until 1945, when ill health prevented him from carrying out his numerous duties and responsibilities, and he requested the appointment of Nolan D. C. Lewis as managing editor. Jelliffe died later that same year. Under the editorship of Lewis and his successors the *Journal* became predominantly, if not entirely, a psychiatric publication, no longer serving as a forum for the publication of papers dealing with neurologic subjects.

ARCHIVES OF NEUROLOGY

In 1917 the Board of Trustees of the American Medical Association (AMA) established a monthly journal, the *Archives of Neurology and Psychiatry,* with the understanding that it would replace the *Journal of Nervous and Mental Disease* as the official organ of the American Neurological Association. The first editorial board consisted of Hugh T. Patrick, Pearce Bailey, Elmer E. Southard, August Hoch, and Theodore H. Weisenburg. The first issue appeared in January 1919. It contained an editorial announcement in which it is stated, "There [is] need for a publication which would keep its readers in touch with the best work in all countries, and which would help to elevate the general standard of knowledge of the nervous system and its disease. . . . The need is for a scientific publication of high ideals which will not only serve the purpose of the research man and technical expert, but which shall also be of immediate practical value to the clinician." Weisenburg was appointed editor-in-chief in 1920 and served in this capacity until his death in 1934. He was succeeded by H. Douglas Singer, who served as editor-in-chief until his death in 1940. He in turn was succeeded by Tracy J. Putnam who served as chief editor from 1940 through 1955. In 1956 Harold G. Wolff was appointed chief editor for neurology and Roy R. Grinker Sr. chief editor for psychiatry. Beginning in 1957 there were separate sections for neurology and psychiatry, continuing under the editorship of Wolff and Grinker, respectively.

Although the *Archives* was the official journal of the American Neurological Association, it dealt with neurology and psychiatry, and there was agitation on the part of members of both specialty groups to have two separate journals. Largely through the efforts of Roland Mackay, Percival Bailey, and Paul Bucy, the Board of Trustees of the AMA finally agreed to this in 1959, and the *Archives of Neurology* and the *Archives of General Psychiatry* were established. The last issue of the combined journal was published in June 1959, completing volume 81, and the first number of the *Archives of Neurology* appeared in July 1959. Wolff continued as chief editor of the *Archives of Neurology* and held this position until his death in 1962. He was succeeded by H. Houston Merritt, who served as chief editor for 9 years, when he retired. On January 1, 1972, Fred Plum assumed the post of chief editor. In 1975 Plum and the entire editorial board of the *Archives of Neurology* resigned because of differences of opinion between them and the editorial offices of the AMA. At the same time the *Archives* ceased to be the official journal of the American Neurological Association. The Board of Trustees of the AMA then appointed Maurice W. Van Allen chief editor, named a new editorial board, and continued the publication as a monthly journal.

NEUROLOGY

One of the first ventures of the American Academy of Neurology, after its establishment in 1948, was the founding of a journal devoted to the specialty. The members expressed the belief that the Academy would develop and prosper only if it had an official publication with which it could be identified. At that time there was no American publication devoted exclusively to neurology. The existing journals dealing with neurology, the *Journal of Nervous and Mental Disease* and the *Archives of Neurology and Psychiatry*, dealt with neurology and psychiatry. A moving force toward the establishment of a neurology journal was Robert Wartenberg, who at that time was professor of neurology at the University of California Medical School in San Francisco. A committee of the Academy consisting of Abe B. Baker (then president of the Academy), Howard D. Fabing, Francis M. Forster, and Adolph L. Sahs (all to be presidents of the Academy) met, made plans for establishing a neurologic journal, and appointed Russell N. DeJong editor-in-chief and Webb Haymaker associate editor. The first editorial board consisted of Raymond D. Adams, Pearce Bailey, Douglas N. Buchanan, Francis M. Forster, Mabel G. Masten, Richard B. Richter, Augustus S. Rose, Alphonse R. Vonderahe, A. Earl Walker, Robert Wartenberg, and Paul I. Yakovlev. The name *Neurology* was adopted for the journal.

The first issue of *Neurology* appeared in January 1951, with the editorial statement, "It seems fitting to assume that for the most effective expression of our aims and accomplishments, we, as neurologists, should have autonomy in publications as well as in teaching, administration, and practice. With this in view, the first issue of *Neurology* is issued under the auspices of the Board of Trustees of the American Academy of Neurology. *Neurology* is intended to be a medium for the prompt publication of articles dealing with the structure, function, and pathology of the nervous system, including the therapeutic aspects of such pathologic states, and to stimulate individual investigation in these various fields." The journal was issued as a bimonthly publication during its first 2 years, but by that time the number of papers submitted was so great that it became necessary to publish it monthly. DeJong continued as editor-in-chief for 26 years. In 1977 he was named founding editor and Lewis P. Rowland was appointed editor-in-chief. Associate editors were Webb Haymaker (1951–1953), Mabel G. Masten (1954–1961), and Kenneth R. Magee (1969–1976). Stanley Fahn was appointed associate editor in 1977.

ANNALS OF NEUROLOGY

After Plum's resignation from the *Archives of Neurology,* he and the American Neurological Association, of which he was at that time the president, made arrangements with Little, Brown and Company of Boston to publish a new journal to be called the *Annals of Neurology* which would be the official journal of the Association as well as of the Child Neurology Society. Plum was named editor, and the original editorial board was the same as that which resigned from the *Archives,* although more members were added later. The first issue was published in January 1977, and it has appeared monthly since that time.

OTHER PUBLICATIONS

Other journals dealing with neurologic material were also published from time to time. Some of them were short-lived, and others were mainly of local interest. Still others dealt with special aspects of neurology or with basic sciences closely allied to neurology. In 1874 George M. Beard established the *Archives of Electrology and Neurology,* which lasted only 2 years. The *Alienist and Neurologist* was founded and edited by Jerome K. Bauduy and C. H. Hughes in St. Louis in 1880 and continued publication for 40 years. William A. Hammond and William G. Morton published three issues of *Neurological Contributions* between 1879 and 1881, and a homeopathic enterprise, the *American Journal of Electrology and Neurology,* edited by John Butler, came out in four numbers between July 1879 and April 1880. Edward C. Spitzka, editor, assisted by Thomas A. McBride and Landon Carter Gray, established the *American Journal of Neurology and Psychiatry* in February 1882. It closed with volume 3 in 1885. James S. Jewell published four numbers of the *Neurological Review* in 1886, but poor health forced him to suspend publication. Thomas A. McBride published the *Review of Insanity and Nervous Diseases* in five volumes between 1890 and 1894. Issues of the *Transactions of the New York Neurological Society* were published in 1894 and 1896. Ira Van Gieson established the *Archives of Neurology and Psychopathology* in 1898, and its publication was terminated in 1900.

Neurographs, published as an "occasional journal" between 1907 and 1915 by William Browning of Brooklyn, contained articles by "men more or less associated with the editor."

The *Bulletin of the Neurological Institute of New York* appeared in 1931 under the editorship of Oliver Strong. Its establishment was largely initiated by Frederick Tilney, and after his death in 1938 publication was suspended. The *Bulletin of the Los Angeles Neurological Society* first appeared in 1936 through the influence of Cyril Courville, Johannes M. Nielsen, and Carl W. Rand. It continues to be published and in later years has been sponsored by the Los Angeles Society of Psychiatry and Neurology and the Southern California Neurosurgical Society. A monthly journal *Diseases of the Nervous System* was founded in 1939 with Titus Harris, professor of neurology and psychiatry at the Medical Branch of the University of Texas in Galveston, as editor. The journal remained a rather small one and from the beginning dealt more with psychiatry than neurology. In 1978 the name was changed to the *Journal of Clinical Psychiatry.*

Of the journals dealing with the basic sciences related to neurology, the *Journal of Comparative Neurology* is the most durable. It was started in 1891 in Cincinnati by Clarence L. Herrick and was transferred to Denison University in Granville, Ohio, the next year. In 1893 Herrick became ill and his brother C. Judson Herrick assumed the editorial duties, which he continued until 1908 when the journal was acquired by the Wistar Institute. He continued to serve as a member of the editorial board until his retirement, when he was named editor emeritus. The 100th volume appeared in 1954, and the journal continues to be published. Other specialty journals are as follows: the *Journal of Neurophysiology* was established by the American Physiological Society in 1938; the *Journal of Neuropathology and Experimental Neurology* was established by the American Association of Neuropathologists in 1942; the *Journal of Neurosurgery* was established in 1944 by the Harvey Cushing Society, which later assumed the name of the American Association of Neurological Surgeons; *Electroencephalography and Clinical Neurophysiology* is an international journal, but Americans have at all times held important posts on its editorial board; the *Journal of Neurochemistry* is also an international journal which first appeared in 1956; *Experimental Neurology* with William F. Windle as editor-in-chief has been published since 1959; *Stroke: A Journal of Cerebral Circulation* was established in 1970 by the American Heart Association; *Surgical Neurology* has been published since 1973 by Paul C. Bucy; *Muscle-Nerve* has been published since 1978; and finally, the *American Journal of Neuroradiology,* official journal of the American Society of Neuroradiology, first appeared in 1980.

The Association for Research in Nervous and Mental Disease was organized in 1920 and has held annual meetings since that time. Each year current research dealing with a single topic of timely interest to either neurology or psychiatry is discussed in detail. The president for the year is an individual who has special interest and experience in the subject under discussion, and the members of the Commission are also specialists in the subject. Most of the papers are presented by members of the Commission and consist of detailed reviews of the various aspects of investigation related to the subject under discussion. *The Proceedings of the Association* are published annually and are important additions to current neurologic and psychiatric literature.

The Transactions of the American Neurological Association appear annually in book form. They contain brief reports of the papers at the annual meeting of the Association as well as minutes of the business meetings. Most, but not all, of the papers presented are published later in more detail in one of the major neurologic journals.

11

Neurology and the Federal Services

American medical education and American medicine as a clinical discipline had their beginnings during the Revolutionary War and the years immediately following it. Neurology as a clinical specialty had its birth during the Civil War and owes its development to the specialized hospitals that were established by Surgeon General William A. Hammond for the treatment of nerve injuries and nervous system diseases as well as to the meticulous studies on the clinical manifestations and treatment of these entities that were carried out in these hospitals by S. Weir Mitchell and his associates.

AMERICAN NEUROLOGY DURING WORLD WAR I

During World War I neurologists and psychiatrists worked together in the study and treatment of nerve injuries and nervous disorders in military personnel in the United States and the European theatre of operations. In 1917 a division of neurology and psychiatry, independent of internal medicine, was established in the office of the Surgeon General of the United States Army. This was organized and directed by a neurologist, Pearce Bailey (17). The physicians in the newly created division were mainly psychiatrists, but neurologists were in charge of most of the hospitals and stations. It was at this time that the term neuropsychiatry came into general usage.

The psychiatrists in the U.S. Army during World War I were recruited largely from state hospital systems and had received their training through the performance of routine duties. They were, largely, hospital administrators with experience in the management of the psychoses but with little training in the treatment of the psychoneuroses and none in the care of patients with organic disorders of the nervous system. The neurologists, on the other hand, were trained in the care of patients with organic diseases of the nervous system, and most had office experience with the care of the psychoneuroses, but they lacked training in the management of the psychoses. Because of these divergent backgrounds and experience, it was deemed necessary to give supplementary training to neurologists and psychiatrists in areas where their experience was deficient. In the military services neurology and psychiatry were united into neuropsychiatry. In spite of the additional training of psychiatrists in the care of organic disease and of neurologists in the management of the psychoses, the war neuroses, or psychoneuroses, proved to be the major medical problem, not only for the neuropsychiatrists but also for physicians in all branches of the service.

Shortly before the end of the war, plans were conceived for establishing a special hospital for the care of patients with nerve injuries and nervous disorders in the Washington, D.C. area, but once discharge from the service was started there were political pressures to hasten the return of veterans to their homes, and plans for the special hospital were canceled. At the end of the war the Division of Neurology and Psychiatry was absorbed into the Division of Medicine and Surgery of the United States Army.

AMERICAN NEUROLOGY DURING WORLD WAR II

During World War II, unlike World War I, the divisions of neuropsychiatry of all the medical departments of the Armed Services as well as all of the administrative posts were headed by psychiatrists (7,15). As in World War I, the war neuroses were again considered to be the major medical problem. This time, however, it was psychiatrists who played the predominant role in their therapy. The neurologists served mainly as consultants to the neuropsychiatric services. Early in 1942, shortly after the United States had entered the war, the neuropsychiatric branch of the Office of the Surgeon General of the Army was elevated to division status, on a level with the divisions of medicine and surgery. Neurology thus became one of the four branches of the Office, and William H. Everts was appointed chief of neurology. Later in the war he was succeeded by Alexander T. Ross.

The organization for the handling of neurosurgical casualties posed difficult problems (12). The principle, adopted by the surgeon general early in the war, that all brain, spinal cord, and peripheral nerve injuries should be treated in base hospitals in the United States caused difficulties as the site of the conflict was thousands of miles away from centers for specialized care. Under Loyal Davis, senior consultant in neurosurgery, assisted by John Scarff and R. Glen Spurling, an attempt was made to have neurology and neurosurgery administratively join in European base hospitals, but this was possible in only a few (12,15).

Specialty units for the care and treatment of peripheral nerve, spinal cord, and brain injuries were established in the European theatre and the continental United States. Stimulated by accomplishments made in these centers, several long-term follow-up studies of neurosurgical wounds were published in monograph form. Among these were Walker and Jablon's observation of the posttraumatic course of service men who developed epilepsy as a result of head wounds (16) and the detailed analysis of the results of surgical therapy for peripheral nerve injuries carried out in specialized centers by Woodhall and Beebee (18).

NEUROLOGY IN THE VETERANS ADMINISTRATION

Prior to 1946 neurologic medicine and research were not recognized by the Veterans Administration (VA) as specific disciplines within the field of medicine. That year, during reorganization of the medical services in the VA, Pearce Bailey Jr., on separation from his neurologic duties at the Philadelphia Naval Hospital, was asked to take charge of the neurologic program that was then under neuropsychiatry in the Division of Medicine and Surgery of the VA, succeeding Howard D. Fabing, who wished to return to the private practice of neurology in Cincinnati (1,2). The reorganization had begun under the direction of two veteran generals of the European theatre of operations, Omar N. Bradley, Administrator, and Paul R. Hawley, Chief Medical Director of the VA. The new leadership was strengthened by the appointment of Paul B. Magnuson, professor of orthopedic surgery at Northwestern University Medical School, as head of the educational and research programs of the VA.

The new medical program included three major policy changes: (a) the Dean's Committee plan, which was designed to bring medicine in the VA into closer association with academic medicine; (b) the location of new VA hospitals in close proximity to medical schools and medical centers; (c) strengthening the clinical and research staffs of the VA hospitals through providing modernized clinical facilities, increased research opportunities, salary inducements, and academic appointments for VA physicians. One of the first actions of the new chief of neurology was the appointment of a medical advisory committee, members of which were selected by the council of the American Neurological Association. Henry A. Riley was asked to be chairman of this committee, and other members were Bernard J. Alpers, R. Foster Kennedy, Lewis J. Pollock, Walter F. Schaller, and Edwin G. Zabriskie. Shortly after the committee was established, H. Houston Merritt was also made a member. The committee met monthly with the chief of neurology.

As a result of the encouragement and support of the new leadership, clinical facilities and research programs expanded rapidly in the medical schools affiliated with VA hospitals. Soon facilities for residency training in neurology became available in many centers throughout the country, and residency training programs were established, expanded, and improved. The support of individual research projects was not an outstanding feature of early policy as the major impetus was directed toward improvement in medical care. The neurology section, however, through the assistance of its civilian consultants, did organize several pilot and demonstration projects involving improvement of medical care for veterans. These included the National Epilepsy Center at Framingham, Massachusetts, under the direction of William G. Lennox; several electroencephalography programs under the supervision of Frederic A. Gibbs; a center for aphasic disorders in Los Angeles under J. M. Nielsen; a center for the study of injuries of the spinal

cord, cauda equina, and peripheral nerves in Chicago under Lewis J. Pollock, and a center in Minneapolis for neurologic rehabilitation under A. B.
Baker and J. R. Brown.

In 1947 the name of the Section of Neuropsychiatry was changed to that of
Psychiatry and Neurology, which gave more autonomy to neurology and
enhanced its prestige. Bailey continued as chief of neurology until 1959,
when he resigned to become director of the newly established National
Institute of Neurological Diseases and Blindness. In 1972 neurology became
a separate service in the VA with Warren V. Huber as director.

NATIONAL INSTITUTE OF NEUROLOGICAL DISEASES
AND BLINDNESS

The establishment of a federally supported national institute for the investigation and treatment of combat injuries to nerves and other diseases of the
nervous system was first proposed by Harvey Cushing toward the end of
World War I, but the rapid discharge of military personnel following the
cessation of hostilities and a general lack of enthusiasm for the project
caused the plans to be dropped. During the late 1940s and early 1950s several
voluntary health agencies concerned with diseases affecting the nervous
system were organized (3,5,11). The first of these was the National Foundation for Infantile Paralysis. Members included friends and admirers of President Franklin D. Roosevelt, and the Foundation was well supported and
endorsed. Other similar agencies followed, the first of which were the National Multiple Sclerosis Society, Muscular Dystrophy Association of
America, United Cerebral Palsy Association, Myasthenia Gravis Foundation, and National Epilepsy League. Others were soon added. Members of
these groups were interested in research and treatment of neurologic diseases and requested federal support. Many active and prominent
neurologists testified before congressional committees to recommend federal funding.

In 1949 the National Multiple Sclerosis Society, through Sylvia Lawry, its
director, and Ralph Strauss, president of its board of directors, solicited the
aid of Senator Charles W. Tobey of New Hampshire, whose daughter had
the disease, in requesting Congress to establish a National Institute for Multiple Sclerosis. This request was not granted, but a year later Senator Tobey,
along with others, petitioned for the establishment of a national institute for
study and treatment of neurologic, visual, and sensory disorders in the National Institutes of Health (NIH), a part of the United States Public Health
Service in the Department of Health, Education and Welfare, and there was
a favorable response. In 1951 the National Institute of Neurological Diseases
and Blindness (NINDB) was established (4–6). This was later to be known,
after the separation of ocular disease and the establishment of the National
Institute for Eye Research, as the National Institute of Neurological and

Communicative Disorders and Stroke. In the fall of 1951, Pearce Bailey was appointed first director of the Institute.

The programs and policies of the NINDB were determined by an Advisory Council consisting of six professionals (neurologic scientists, otologists, ophthalmologists, audiologists, etc.), six public-spirited citizens, and *ex officio* members from the Department of Defense and the Veterans Administration. The Council also reviewed all research grant, training grant, and fellowship applications.

During its early years the NINDB was limited in its activities because of budgetary restrictions. In 1951 its budget was $1,250,000, mainly transferred funds from the National Institute of Mental Health and the Division of Research Grants. In 1952 the budget was $1,992,300. This low budget was due in part to the fact that the representatives from the voluntary health agencies testifying before Congress were not united in their efforts and in part to the fact that the requests for assistance for the investigation of neurologic disorders did not have the emotional appeal of cancer, heart disease, and mental health. Soon after his appointment, the director called a meeting of neurologic scientists and representatives from the voluntary groups to discuss means for organizing a concerted program for neurologic research. As a result the Committee for Research in Neurological Disorders was organized, with A. B. Baker as chairman. He was succeeded in 1970 by Paul C. Bucy. Once this committee was organized and its members began testifying before Congress, the NINDB was given its own identifiable appropriation. In 1953 the budget was $4,500,000, and it grew to over $125,000,000 in 1975.

The first grants awarded by the NINDB were for research, but soon funds became available for graduate training programs for teachers and investigators. Fellowships were awarded for training in the allied disciplines of neuropathology, neurochemistry, electroencephalography, neuro-ophthalogy, and related disciplines (8).

With the completion of the NIH's Clinical Center in 1953, space was allocated there for the NINDB. In May of that year G. Milton Shy and Maitland Baldwin took up their duties as directors of the medical and surgical intramural programs of the NINDB. Intramural and extramural research programs and clinical and basic science investigations were supported by the NINDB, as well as collaborative, multidisciplinary, multi-institutional, and field investigations. It also sponsored seminars, symposia, and conferences dealing with widespread neurology-related subjects ranging from basic research to clinical neurologic education. American neurology would not have risen to its present peak had it not been for the NINDB and the institutes it spawned.

In 1959 Bailey resigned as director to join another research program, and he was succeeded by Richard L. Masland, who had been appointed assistant director in 1958. He in turn was succeeded in 1968 by William F. MacNichol Jr., who served until 1973 (9,10). In June 1974 Donald B. Tower became director (14). In 1975 the NINDB celebrated its 25th anniversary with the publication of a three-volume historical survey and scientific review of its important contributions (13).

REFERENCES

1. Bailey, P. (1946): Plans in progress for the care of neurological patients under the Veterans Administration. *Trans. Am. Neurol. Assoc.,* 71:7–9.
2. Bailey, P. (1947): Program for the activation of neurology under the Veterans Administration. *J.A.M.A.,* 134:1283–1284.
3. Bailey, P. (1949): The present outlook of neurology in the United States. *J. Assoc. Am. Med. Coll.,* 24:214–215.
4. Bailey, P. (1953): America's first national neurologic institute. *Neurology (Minneap.),* 3:321–325.
5. Bailey, P. (1975): Government organization of neurological research and development in the Veterans Administration and the National Institute of Neurological Disease and Blindness. In: *Centennial Anniversary Volume of the American Neurological Association 1875–1975,* edited by D. Denny-Brown, A. S. Rose, and A. L. Sahs, pp. 509–531. Springer, New York.
6. Bailey, P. (1975): The National Institute of Neurological Diseases and Blindness: Origins, founding and early years (1950–1959). In: *The Basic Neurosciences, Vol. 1: The Nervous System: A Three Volume Work Commemorating the Twenty-fifth Anniversary of the National Institute of Neurological and Communicative Disorders and Stroke,* edited by R. O. Brady, pp. xi–xxxii. Raven Press, New York.
7. Glass, A. J., and Bernucci, R. J. (1966): *Neuropsychiatry in World War II, Vol. I: Zone of the Interior.* U.S. Government Printing Office, Washington, D.C.
8. Goldstein, M. (1975): The National Institute of Neurological and Communicative Disorders and Stroke: manpower recruitment and training programs (1950–1975). In: *The Basic Neurosciences, Vol. 1: The Nervous System: A Three Volume Work Commemorating the Twenty-fifth Anniversary of the National Institute of Neurological and Communicative Disorders and Stroke,* edited by R. O. Brady, pp. liii–lvii. Raven Press, New York.
9. MacNichol, E. F., Jr.: The National Institute of Neurological Diseases and Stroke (1968–1973). In: *The Basic Neurosciences, Vol. 1: The Nervous System: A Three Volume Work Commemorating the Twenty-fifth Anniversary of the National Institute of Neurological and Communicative Disorders and Stroke,* edited by R. O. Brady, pp. xicii–lii. Raven Press, New York.
10. Masland, R. L. (1975): The National Institute of Neurological Diseases and Blindness: development and growth (1960–1968). In: *The Basic Neurosciences, Vol. 1: The Nervous System: A Three Volume Work Commemorating the Twenty-fifth Anniversary of the National Institute of Neurological and Communicative Disorders and Stroke,* edited by R. O. Brady, pp. xxxiii–xivi. Raven Press, New York.
11. Merritt, H. H. (1975): The development of neurology in the past fifty years. In: *Centennial Anniversary Volume of the American Neurological Association 1875–1975,* edited by D. Denny-Brown, A. S. Rose, and A. L. Sahs, pp. 3–10. Springer, New York.
12. Spurling, R. G., Woodhall, B., and McGetridge, E. N. (1958): *Surgery in World War II: Neurosurgery.* U.S. Government Printing Office, Washington, D.C.
13. Tower, D. B. (editor-in-chief) (1975): *The Nervous System; A Three Volume Work Commemorating the Twenty-fifth Anniversary of the National Institute of Neurological and Communicative Disorders and Stroke; Vol. 1: The Basic Neurosciences; Vol. 2, The Clinical Neurosciences; Vol. 3, Human Communication and Its Disorders.* Raven Press, New York.
14. Tower, D. B. (1975): Introduction. In: *The Basic Neurosciences, Vol. 1: The Nervous System: A Three Volume Work Commemorating the Twenty-fifth Anniversary of the National Institute of Neurological and Communicative Disorders and Stroke,* edited by R. O. Brady, pp. xvii–xx. Raven Press, New York.

15. Walker, A. E. (1975): The contribution of neurology to the military services in the last fifty years. In: *Centennial Anniversary Volume of the American Neurological Association 1875–1975,* edited by D. Denny-Brown, A. S. Rose, and A. L. Sahs, pp. 532–542. Springer, New York.
16. Walker, A. E., and Jablon, S. (1961): *A Follow-up Study of Head Wounds in World War II.* Veterans Administration Medical Monograph. United States Government Printing Office, Washington, D.C.
17. Weisenburg, T. H. (1924): Military history of the American Neurological Association. In: *Semicentennial Anniversary Volume, American Neurological Association (1875–1924),* pp. 262–310. Boyd Printing Co., New York.
18. Woodhall, B., and Beebee, G. W. (1956): *Peripheral Nerve Regeneration: Follow-up Study of 3,655 Injuries.* U.S. Government Printing Office, Washington, D.C.

Subject Index